Staff Development
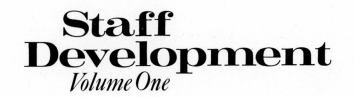
Volume One

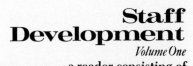

Staff
Development
Volume One
a reader consisting of
nineteen articles especially selected
by The Journal of Nursing Administration
Editorial Staff.

First edition, second printing

Library of Congress Catalog Card Number: 75-3506
International Standard Book Number: 0-913654-08-6

Type set by WILLIAMS GRAPHIC SERVICE, INC.

Manufactured in The United States of America
by WILLIAM BYRD PRESS, Richmond, Virginia

Contents

Guidelines for Organizing Inservice Education

by Naomi D. Medearis and Elda S. Popiel

Naomi D. Medearis obtained an M.A. in education from the University of Denver College of Arts and Sciences and an M.B.A. in personnel and industrial relations from the Graduate School of Business Administration at New York University. Currently she is an educational consultant and vice president of Associates for Continuing Education, Inc., consulting with health, business, educational and religious organizations. At the time this article was written she was associate professor (Continuing Education Programs) at the University of Colorado School of Nursing.

Elda S. Popiel, R.N., M.S., is Professor Emeritus, Continuing Education Programs, University of Colorado School of Nursing, and presently consultant in continuing education. Mrs. Popiel earned her B.S. in nursing at Avila College and her M.S. in nursing at the University of Colorado. This article is reprinted from JONA, November-December, 1973.

Guidelines for Organizing Inservice Education is an article concerned with the roles of the director of nursing service and the inservice educator as they develop the inservice education program for their health agency

The articulation of their roles and their shared responsibilities are delineated as are the steps to be taken to develop a dynamic and successful inservice program. Emphasis is placed on a learning model which demonstrates the teaching-learning process and the training cycle. Cooperation, collaboration, and a sharing in program planning, implementation, and evaluation with the staff participants is discussed.

The need for inservice education in health agencies emerges from the phenomenon of change—change in what is known about man and how he functions in health and illness, change in the ways people meet the challenge of crisis and daily living, change in the patterns of care and what the public expects in health care, change in health legislation, change in the scientific knowledge and discoveries and change in the objectives, organization, and financing of health services. Health agencies are becoming aware of their responsibility in the field of inservice for their employees and are appointing specific individuals to direct the inservice program. Many of these appointees are nurses. Often these nurses have had no formal education which would prepare them for the inservice education assignment. Knowledge about how adults learn, how to assess and validate educational needs, writing behavioral objectives, planning teaching-learning experiences in order to reach the objectives, and evaluation and implementation of inservice programs is comparatively lacking in the educational background of the majority of the nurses who have the responsibility for inservice programs.

For the inservice program to be successful and dynamic, it must be designed as a learning model and demonstrate the teaching-learning process and the training cycle (Fig. 1). The inservice educator becomes a part of this model

and is a co-learner along with those she teaches. Inservice education programs are not a do-it-yourself operation or a ''one-man'' show; they must be shared programs in planning as well as in implementation and evaluation.

The director of nursing service and the administration of the health agency have a shared responsibility in the program, as do the inservice director and the employees. All must be involved in a variety of ways for the program to be dynamic, challenging, and successful. Guidelines can be developed to provide the structure for a firm foundation from which to operate.

To use the guidelines in a vital way, an open communication system is needed. This quality and climate of openness is a constant yet everchanging demand on the relationship of the inservice educator and the director of nursing. This trust develops through open discussions of expectations, values, ideas, strategies, feelings, and perceptions of each other's role and the use of guidelines. Differences not openly dealt with in these areas of work

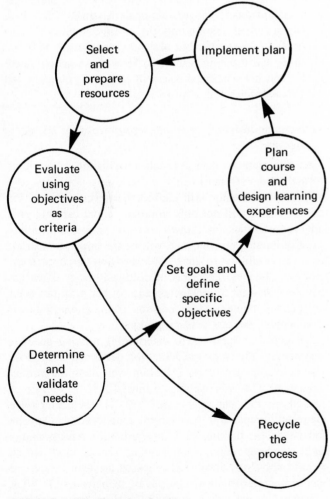

FIGURE 1 The Training Cycle

Adapted from *Learning to Work in Groups,* page 38. Matthew B. Miles. Teachers College. Columbia University, N.Y. 1959.

carry with them the seeds of threat, resentment, a sense of futility, distrust, and a critical dissipation of energy.

Creating a style of giving, taking, and sharing demands honesty, respect, caring, and a nonevaluative stance. One person cannot do it alone. When this atmosphere is present it will permit creative collaboration in planning inservice, and the model of this openness will filter through nursing service in many different ways and at surprisingly different levels. It will change the image of inservice.

The other vital component of an open communication system built by the director of nursing and inservice educator is listening ability and time. To listen with an acceptance of the person and an openness to hear the total message demands strict discipline of self. A conscious effort to build in a feedback norm supports this open communication system and assists it in achieving a state of equilibrium.

An approach built on this foundation within nursing service will create a climate geared to growth rather than to ''fixing up people'' and ''correcting mistakes.''

A clear contract or working agreement between the nursing director and the inservice educator will need to be made. At regular intervals, both need to check out how well this contract is being met. This practice will release the energy to renew the efforts of both to offer a meaningful, practical, and timely program. Only by conscientiously and openly building this ongoing relationship can the guidelines be useful.

GUIDELINES FOR THE NURSING DIRECTOR

Of paramount importance in the success of any inservice program is a participating philosophy concerned about the development of every individual and faith that employees will make the right decisions if given the necessary information and support. Emphasis must be placed on the release of human potential rather than on the control of human behavior which ''in reality means developing people to do a good job rather than a minimum job.''[1] Everyone concerned must believe and work toward mutual trust, openness of communication, a general attitude of helpfulness and cooperation, and a willingness to accept responsibility. The participating philosophy must encompass the belief that learning activities will be based on real educational needs and interests of the employees. The program will be determined by a group that is representative of all participants, and there will be involvement of all members in making and carrying out decisions.

No inservice program will be successful without the full cooperation and support of the nursing service director of the health agency. This support must be tangible, intangible, and consistent. ''An organization's most effective instrument of influence is its own behavior.''[2] An organization's behavior is molded by the administration

3

and establishes the climate in the organization. The provision of a structure which allows the nursing staff to try out new ideas, skills, and knowledge and to take risks and experiment is essential. It is the responsibility of the director to see that the goals set up by the inservice director are consistent with those of nursing service and the health agency. Assistance and support in making the program relevant to the educational needs of the health personnel as related to the health care needs of the consumers of care becomes a specific responsibility of the director.

The nursing director must expect the inservice education director to initiate programs and to be accountable for the programs designed and implemented. Because of these expectations the nursing director does not "saddle" the director with duties that do not pertain to the inservice program.

Tangible support is most often exemplified in the amount of funds allotted in the nursing service budget to the inservice program. The provision of clerical assistance, office space, conference space, and teaching aids is also a concrete form of support for the inservice director.

The nursing director's creative efforts in communicating her expectations and in freeing people for full involvement in the inservice sessions will allow health personnel to concentrate their energies on the learning situation. The end result will be improved health care and satisfied employees attempting to work at their maximum potential.

GUIDELINES FOR THE INSERVICE EDUCATOR

Define for herself her role as inservice director and test it continuously with clients–administrators, staff personnel, colleagues, auxiliary personnel.

Traditionally, the inservice educator has been asked to or has assumed responsibility for updating nursing procedures, staging fire drills, planning safety programs for all personnel, and many other programs not relevant to nursing care.

The inservice director needs to become aware of the expectations she has for herself and those others hold for her. As the person charged with the overall inservice responsibility, she should determine *what is and what is not* inservice. If she knows where she is going, others will be able to adjust their expectations of her and of her approach to inservice.

For successful patient-centered and employee-centered nursing education, she will need to identify and sell her priorities to her clients. Her time and energy need to be channeled, and she should assume major responsibility for this.

In defining her role the director of inservice should ask herself, (1) How did I get this job? (2) Do I really want it? (3) What is expected of me? (4) What do I consider to be inservice? (5) How do I find out what people really

need and want to know to do their jobs more effectively? (6) How do I get people to try out new things? (7) How do I set priorities? (8) What risks am I willing to take? (9) What ideas do other health personnel have that I can draw on to improve nursing performance? (10) How can I plan inservice that is meaningful to personnel in nursing service—people at all levels? (11) How can I get the right people "involved" in inservice training? (12) What criteria do I use to measure the effectiveness of the inservice program? (13) What is my reward as inservice director? (14) What do I see happening in inservice five years from now?

As she defines her role and determines her responsibilities, the director will find relevant data in her day-to-day work with staff. Head nurse meetings will provide opportunities to "tune-in" on their concerns as supervisors of patient care. Organizing special task forces to assess needs and serve as planners for specific clinical nursing areas extends the inservice role and provides data for inservice programming. Physicians, x-ray personnel, and physical, occupational, and recreational therapists who share in patient care enrich not only the inservice educator's perception of patient care, but also provide relevant and vital planning and teaching resources. How these people relate to her and her perceived role will help her to clearly and realistically define her own role.

Determine training needs and set priorities for inservice programs.

As she gathers data through observation, interviews (formal and informal), and written questionnaires the inservice coordinator will define the specific needs for training which will not only improve patient care but provide opportunities for growth and prevention of obsolescence of nursing personnel. It will be the inservice instructor's responsibility to make the decision on how these needs will be met. The array of needs will be so extensive that she will want to seek acceptance of her priorities from key people, namely those persons from whom she will need support and active participation.

A significant approach to determining training needs is to systematically study the actual job performance of those who deliver patient care. (1) How well does the patient understand what's happening to him? (2) How well coordinated is the patient's care? (3) Is each employee adequately prepared to perform his functions? (4) Does he understand the nursing care standards? (5) Are there any such standards defined in nursing service and within specific units? (6) How well prepared are team leaders to handle the interpersonal relations of their team? (7) What resources are not being utilized? (8) How are nurses prepared for supervisory and acting positions? (9) How does inservice education relate to these problems? Somehow, the inservice director will need to find answers for these

issues as she works with the nursing personnel.

She may well ask, "How can one person possibly deal with all of this?" One person can't, this is where the next guideline fits in.

Determine the areas for decentralized and centralized inservice programming.

The inservice director will seek to validate with nurse colleagues the fact that a professional nurse includes in her expertise two vital functions—that of teaching and that of supervising members of her staff. She will check out their feelings about their personal competence in these two areas, and involve them in identifying what needs their personnel have to improve performance and how to provide the teaching and coaching to accomplish this. In the process of assessing the needs of their staff they will discover the knowledge and skills they need to handle this phase of their jobs more efficiently and effectively. They will also begin to discover that this approach will build confidence and trust within their unit. As a result the integration of needs and the development of skills to teach and supervise begin to evolve. This process of cooperative planning and programming greatly reduces the threat to the professional nurse and creates a relationship of interdependence which utilizes the resources of both the inservice educator and the nurse-supervisor. It also provides a pattern for realistic inservice education in which on-the-job orientation and training has most impact on results.[3]

Centralize training programs where a common body of knowledge, a special or limited skill, or an overall attitude is the focal point of training.

The premises of "training for training's sake," or "I have a good film," or "Dr. Williams would give a good lecture for us at our next inservice meeting," or "We need a program on theft because things are missing on the third floor" are no longer valid approaches to justify the abandonment of patients under the guise of inservice education.

The inservice educator should raise the questions of why, who, when, and how in the process of making the decisions regarding an inservice program. Using this approach will enable the inservice educator and her committees to tailor an inservice program to the educational needs of the staff involved in the training.

GUIDELINES TO THE TEACHING-LEARNING PROCESS USING THE TRAINING CYCLE

Inservice training has as its primary purpose the discovery and development of attitudes and behavior in such a way that the mission and objectives of the health agency are met and the employee's needs for self-worth, growth, and satisfaction are significantly met in the organization.

The integration of organizational and personal goals within an inservice program is a basic goal for each learning activity.

Using this systems approach, the process of planning specific, realistic, and needed inservice programs can be made manageable and measurable.

Determine and validate training needs.

Training needs can be determined by gathering data from a variety of sources and validated in several ways: first, by interviewing. If the individuals to be trained are interviewed, either formally or informally, an assessment of their knowledge and skill in the area under study will yield vital data on where to begin, what the trainee has going for him, and his attitude toward what he does on his job. Second, the inservice educator can draw on her own and others' guided observations of the performance of nursing functions. This involves constant study of the kind of health care given patients and their families. A third source of data is found in the incident reports and performance evaluations of employees. Using these data, the inservice director can order her training needs and determine priorities for inservice programming. The fourth vital area is validating her perception of these composite needs and priorities with her nursing colleagues and administration. This involvement builds in not only awareness of the direction of future inservice programs, but a beginning degree of ownership in the inservice program itself.

Set goals and objectives for a sequence of programming on a long-range and short-range basis.

Attention to continuity, reinforcement, and timing is essential in building a comprehensive picture of just how inservice education is going to be implemented. Here again the initiative is the inservice director's; however, if she works with an advisory committee, the results will be worth the effort. Members of the advisory committee should be thoughtfully selected and be the subject of another article.

Planning the course or session and designing the learning experience.

The planning and designing of learning experiences challenges the inservice coordinator to draw on the rich methodologies of adult education and action-learning styles. Since the primary goal of inservice is more than giving information and is geared to changing the way a person performs, thinks, or feels, the plan calls for skill in "helping the student" to integrate the new knowledge or skill into his immediate experience and stimulate him to set future learning goals for himself. Role playing, simulated games, small group work, alone time, lectures,

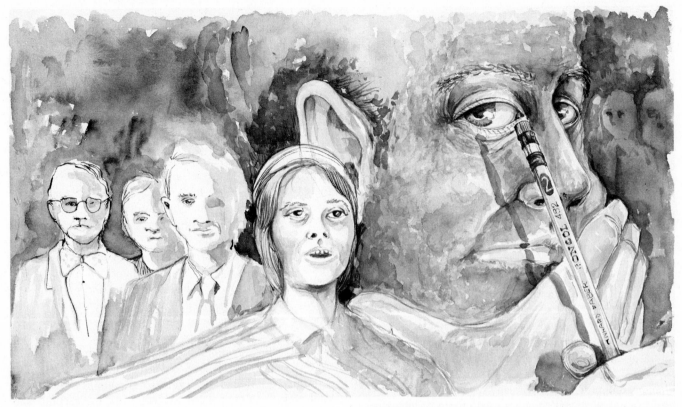

independent study, pilot projects, and other methods facilitate the involvement and response of the "total person" to the learning situation.

Implementation of the plan.

The next phase centers around designing the curriculum. Content requirements, learning experiences, and expectations of the participant provide input for the program outline and schedule. In this area the inservice educator needs to tap the wealth of data in theories of learning and the methodologies that capitalize on the unique attributes of the adult learner. Designing for active involvement of the learner is both an art and a science.

Select resources.

After the formulation of the overall plan, selecting competent resource people becomes the next concern. Criteria for this selection is threefold: (1) Ability to adapt professional knowledge and expertise to "layman-type audiences." This ability is essential if the resource person is to be understood and his expertise utilized. (2) Ability to adapt "expertise" to stated training objectives. Unless the resource person has been given a well-developed set of objectives, he will need to fall back on his own experience and perception of what the participant needs to know. (3) Ability to listen to and respect the knowledge and experience of the participants. The assessment of this quality places a special responsibility on the training director. If the resource person believes and communicates respect

and builds on it, he will be an acceptable resource as far as participants are concerned.

Organizing the program will mean carefully preparing resource people and trainees to work together in the course. Resource people will need well prepared answers to questions like these:

Why me? How do I fit in with the overall program?
What do you want from me?
What are the people like that you want me to work with?
What will they want to know?
What do you expect to happen when it's over?

These questions need to be answered for participants in a training program, also. They too provide a reservoir of resources that need to be tapped. To tap reservoirs, however, participants will need to know honestly what is in it for them. By getting in touch with this data, motivation of the participant has a chance of happening. He is freed to become involved and to accept the change that learning creates and demands.

Evaluation.

The next phase is to evaluate the inservice program, which in effect means measuring the degree of change in the participant's knowledge, ability, and skill, Clearly stated objectives help measure the degree of change in performance. Pretests and post-tests measure changes in knowledge. Guided observation over a period of time will result in assessing the ability of the participant to integrate the learning in the performance of his job.

Recycling The Training Process

The last phase is to start all over again. Based on validation of new needs which emerge from the evaluation process and changes which have evolved during the intervening time, recycling of the program begins.

All of these phases in the planning process involve others. This is true whether the inservice program is decentralized or centralized. To clarify this approach to inservice programming, a case in point is offered.

Decentralized Inservice

The case centers around a head nurse, Mrs. Laura Williams, in an outpatient clinic of a hospital. She had been employed as head nurse for 10 years. A year earlier she had attended an intensive 4-week course in leadership development. With the traineeship came the opportunity to extend her leadership skills by planning and using an 8-hour consultation with the consultant of her choice.

The challenge to use the consultation came in a roundabout way. And here began the chain of events that highlighted the process of planning an inservice program by using the guidelines outlined.

The head nurse section was floundering in the tradition of many well-meaning groups. They were seeking some kind of new direction and came up with two alternatives. They first approached a former faculty member of the school of nursing to serve as an advisor to the group. The person approached refused; she was involved in research for nursing service. The group did not move to the second alternative—approaching the inservice educator for guidance. As a result the head nurse group lost what little cohesion it had and seemed immobilized to develop goals or aims.

It was at this point that Mrs. Williams began to realize her own personal responsibility as a member of the group. She had an opportunity to suggest a potential resource to the group, her 8 hours of consultation service. She called the program coordinator in continuing education to follow-up data she needed for utilizing her consultation. An appointment was set up with the coordinator, and the sequence of the training cycle began to happen; the result, a day-long workshop.

Mrs. Williams' awareness of the need of her group for greater cohesion was validated. She went back to the next section meeting of head nurses with her offer to share her consultation time. The group had never had this kind of experience and agreed to explore the possibilities. Mrs. Williams asked them to come up with the problems they were experiencing in their own sections. When these were reported at the next section meeting of head nurses, it was a logical step to form objectives for the workshop. Their problems:

1. The staff involved were unable to work as a cohesive group.
2. They were unable to communicate with one another.
3. The staff did not feel they knew one another and, therefore, could not trust one another.
4. They lacked knowledge about the group process and the responsibilities of the members as a working group.

To make a choice as to which approach the group wanted to take, a special bring-your-own-lunch meeting was planned. The following ideas emerged from this planning session.

Group dynamics and new ways of looking at the group were selected as the overall concern. Defined objectives were stated:

Objective I. To help each member of the group to work effectively as part of a cohesive group.

a. How do we succeed in creating and maintaining the interest of the group?
b. How can division of interest be prevented?
c. Once a common interest is established, where do we go?
d. How do we go about accomplishing the goal of getting our ideas across to administration?

Objective II. To help each member of the group to function better in a changing situation.

a. How can head nurses prepare themselves for changes which are inevitable? (Some nurses had expressed feelings of antagonism when news of the phasing out of supervisors was received through the "grapevine" well ahead of the official channel notification.)
b. "Everyone tells us that we can be a powerful group," said one nurse. Do we really have influence? How do we go about becoming effective? Is this fact or fiction?

Objective III. To learn to examine ourselves as individuals considering the total person.

a. Some of those present stated that they experienced "hang-ups" with those in a supervisory or staff level but did not feel this way on a peer level.
b. A suggestion was made that perhaps some psychodrama be included in the program to help achieve Objective III.

The next decisions the head nurse group made in planning their own learning experience was to use a training laboratory method rather than an instrumented approach. The dates were determined by the group, the names of resource people were presented, and the group made the choice. Behind each decision was the intent to gain real participation in the decision-making process and to provide a model of the process so that it could be used in other recycling problem-solving workshops.

The resource person was selected and carefully briefed by Mrs. Williams in terms of the head nurse section's process of developing the plan and the specific objectives to be met. The location, meals, manner of dress—all of these decisions were shared with the section heads, which facilitated the climate for building the workshop.

One month after the program was completed, the process of evaluation followed. The participants were asked to give critiques of the experience. Using the specific objectives as the framework, the resource group made open-ended evaluations based on the perceptions of the participants.

The overall result of this inservice was the beginning of a sound organizational approach which greatly facilitated role interpretation of the head nurse as a result of the "inevitable change" mentioned earlier.

In summary, the new skills the inservice educator of today needs evolve around people-skills. The technical skills can be built on the literature and the special audio-visual resource expertise available. But there is no way to avoid the demanding discipline of building inservice on clear-cut guidelines with a keen awareness of sequencing activities clearly relevant to inservice goals and priorities. It is not a job for a loner!

REFERENCES

1. Knowles, M. *The Modern Practice of Adult Education.* Association Press, New York, 1970, p. 61.
2. Herzberg, F. One More Time: How Do You Motivate Employees? *Harvard Business Review*, January-February 1968.
3. Miles, M. B. *Learning to Work in Groups.* Bureau of Publications, Teacher's College, Columbia University, New York, 1959, p. 38.

BIBLIOGRAPHY

Curtis, F. S., Darragh, R. M., Fancher, J. E., Ingmire, A. E., Lesnan, V. B., Orwig, B. I., Popiel, E. S., Shores, W. L. *Continuing Education in Nursing.* WICHE, Boulder, Co., 1969.

Herzberg, F. One More Time: How Do You Motivate Employees? *Harvard Business Review* 46(1): 55–62.

Knowles, M. S. *The Modern Practice of Adult Education.* Association Press, New York, 1970.

Lambertson, E. C. Inservice Education for Emergency Nursing Service. *The Nursing Clinics of North America* 2:237–243, 1967.

Leonard, G. B. *Education and Ecstacy.* Dell Publishing Co., Inc., New York, 1968.

Luft, J. *Group Processes, An Introduction to Group Dynamics.* The National Press, Palo Alto, California, 1963.

Mager, R. F. *Developing Attitudes Toward Learning.* Fearon Publishers, Palo Alto, California, 1968.

Mager, R. F. *Preparing Instructional Objectives.* Fearon Publishers, Palo Alto, California, 1962.

McGregor, D. *The Human Side of Enterprise.* McGraw-Hill Book Company, Inc., New York, 1960.

Nylen, D., Mitchell, J. R. and Stout, A. *Handbook of Staff Development.* Stephenson Lithograph, Inc., Washington, D.C., 1967.

Popiel, E. The Many Facets of Continuing Education in Nursing. *Journal of Nursing Education* 8:1:3–13.

Smith, R. G., Jr. *The Development of Training Objectives.* HumBRO Bulletin II. George Washington University, Alexandria, Virginia, 1964.

Swansburg, R. C. *Inservice Education.* G. P. Putnam's Sons, New York, 1968.

Education for Quality Care

by Marjorie Moore Cantor

Marjorie Moore Cantor, R.N., Ph.D., is associate director of nursing, staff and program development, University of Iowa Hospitals and Clinics. A graduate in nursing from the University of Nebraska, Dr. Cantor received her Master's degree in child welfare research at the University of Iowa where she later earned her Ph.D. in educational psychology.

She has been affiliated with the University of Iowa since 1950 when she was associate in preventive psychiatry on a child welfare research project. Since that time she has served as instructor in nursing, assistant professor of nursing, acting chairman of medical and surgical nursing and assistant professor of nursing in the graduate program. This article is reprinted from JONA, January-February, 1973. It was originally part of a series dealing with the Joint Commission on Accreditation of Hospitals standards for nursing services.

It hardly seems necessary to emphasize to nurses the need for inservice education for the members of a hospital's nursing staff. That the nursing profession assumes considerable responsibility for providing continuing education is amply demonstrated by the amount of literature existing on the subject, by the number of continuing education programs being offered, and by the proliferation of educational materials that are available and used. In addition, several organizations and at least one journal (*The Journal of Continuing Education in Nursing*) is devoted to the problems of inservice and continuing education for nursing personnel.

Even if the need for such educational activities and programs were not continually being called to our attention by journal articles, conference announcements, etc., an awareness of the need would be forced upon us by the problems faced in present-day nursing departments. There was a time when most hospitals could depend on the services of registered nurses whose education ended upon graduation. The activities called for on the job were precisely those for which training was provided prior to graduation. Today, in contrast, the new graduate is typically not prepared to move into a position on a nursing staff without receiving special preparation geared to the particular group of patients whose care she will be responsible for providing. Educational programs producing registered nurses can, in most cases, no longer provide complete preparation for effective on-the-job functioning. Increasingly, nursing departments are finding it necessary to supply further training, focusing specifically on the job being filled by the new graduate.

In addition to registered nurses, other types of health personnel are joining nursing staffs for the first time. The licensed practical nurse is, perhaps, better prepared for the duties she will assume than are other personnel, but typically exposure to a certain amount of content will nonetheless be required to prepare her for the responsibilities she will assume. Aides and orderlies for the most part come completely untrained for their jobs. Their participation in a preservice training program is invariably necessary before they can engage in any nursing care activities.

Induction programs are required, then, for all types of personnel who are members of a hospital's nursing staff. In addition, there exists the never-ending job of updating skills and knowledge to keep staff members abreast of the rapid changes occurring in the field generally and of new programs introduced into their own departments. One could hardly quarrel with the assertion that formal planning for educational needs is a necessity in a well-regulated nursing department.

There is no doubt that Standard V is well accepted by most nursing personnel. But there is reason to be concerned about the philosophy that seems to be directing much of the activity related to the implementation of this standard. Unfortunately the wording of Standard V encourages emphasis on the *educational process itself* rather than on the *reason* for the process—namely, the need to improve the quality of nursing care given patients.

The standard states: "There shall be continuing training programs and *educational opportunities* for the *development of nursing personnel*" [italics mine]. I feel it necessary to take issue with the words italicized in this quoted statement. The implication seems clear that a department is responsible for providing opportunities for its personnel so as to further *their own development*.

It seems to me that if certain educational experiences are necessary to insure the giving of proper care to patients, then the educational program in question should be thought of as comprising a *requirement,* not an "opportunity." The decision as to whether or not personnel should be exposed to this kind of learning experience should not be left to the discretion of the prospective learner. In addition, if the content involved in a learning program does not eventually contribute either directly or indirectly to the welfare of the patient, but simply serves to enhance the personal "development" of the staff member, one might question the right of the department to arrange for the subsidization of such opportunities by the sources that pay for the patient care provided within the institution.

It might be argued that any educational experience is likely to produce patient benefits and that such experiences will necessarily lead staff members to devise ways of improving the welfare of patients. Underlying such an argument is the assumption that education will always necessarily result in "good," and that attendance at workshops, conferences, and speeches on nursing topics can be depended upon as means for improving nursing care. Many nurses believe that a major function of the nursing department is to provide opportunities for individual professional development of its staff members under the assumption that any benefits the staff will derive will eventually enhance the care given to patients.

If one is to determine the extent to which the educational program of a given nursing department is actually contributing effectively to the quality of nursing care,

four crucial sets of questions must be answered. These questions are concerned with the major factors that affect the development and implementation of a useful educational program.

The first factor relates to the philosophy of the individuals responsible for an educational program and how clearly the function served by the program has been identified. The second is concerned with the way educational needs are determined, with particular emphasis on *who* determines them. The third consideration focuses on the extent to which the educational methods chosen are appropriate for the skills to be acquired and efficient in terms of expenditure of time, effort, and resources. The final factor pertains to the criteria to be used in evaluating the effectiveness of a program.

Phrased as questions, the four considerations are as follows:

1. How is the function of inservice education viewed in relation to the other activities required for the provision of patient care? Is staff education seen as a means to an end, or is it treated as *the* end?

2. How and by whom are the educational needs of staff members determined? Are the individuals most qualified to determine the form patient care should take and to evaluate the quality of such care also those who determine the nature of staff education needs?

3. On what basis were the particular educational methods used chosen? Are the methods appropriate to the skills and knowledge to be achieved, and are they economical in terms of expenditure of time, effort, and resources?

4. How is the effectiveness of the educational program evaluated? On the basis of opinions solicited from the recipients of the program? On the basis of the nature of the program's content? Or on the basis of the quality of patient care subsequently given by those participating in the program?

In giving rank to these four sets of considerations, the writer placed evaluation last because the evaluation process is necessarily a terminal one. It will be argued, however, that the *planning* for evaluation should occur at the outset of the development of an educational program, for reasons to be discussed later. The remainder of this paper is devoted to a consideration of each of the four sets of questions listed above.

HOW IS THE FUNCTION OF INSERVICE EDUCATION VIEWED?

The philosophy of the hospital, the department, and persons responsible for educational programs will greatly influence the effectiveness of such programs. If an educational program is seen as something that exists for its own sake, then it is not likely to be evaluated with patient welfare as the focus of concern. Rather, it is apt to be

assessed for the glamour of its content or for its popularity with staff members who have their own personal objectives for a hospital inservice educational program.

It is not unusual for those responsible for a hospital's educational program to view it as an enterprise having a status different from that accorded the daily work of the staff. In this vein, Tosiello[1] has suggested that inservice education should not be controlled by the decisions of a service-oriented authority. He expresses concern that "where prepared educators are employed for this specific task, the noneducational purposes of the agency sometimes stifle them." Such a view, in my opinion, encourages one to emphasize a program rather than its purpose.

This tendency to emphasize program over purpose is apt to be especially strong in situations in which there exist special inservice education units or departments. It is natural for individuals to want their work to be regarded as important by both themselves and others. The main focus of the work of the hospital is, or at least should be, patient care. This being the case, the work of an inservice education unit must be regarded as having an auxiliary character. Under the circumstances, it is understandable that educators might seek to enhance the prestige of their jobs by exaggerating the importance of education for its own sake, thereby creating particularly difficult problems if the service staff see the programs as activities to participate in only if one has some time to spare. Staff members may accept the premise that inservice programs are worthwhile, but at the same time they may tend to view them as extra benefits that must be foregone when service areas are busy. Under such conditions, the main job of the individuals responsible for education becomes one of motivating individuals to attend programs or to provide programs that are acclaimed by the staff.

If education is seen as just one part of a total nursing program to provide quality care to patients, the emphasis will be less on the program itself and more on what the program achieves. Under such conditions, educational programs are not likely to exist as nearly independent entities and continued when they are not effective in helping to maintain or improve the quality of care given to patients.

HOW AND BY WHOM ARE THE EDUCATIONAL NEEDS DETERMINED?

It seems reasonable to assume that staff educational needs should be determined by ascertaining what knowledge is required to make quality nursing care possible and, further, that the individuals best equipped to make this assessment are those nurses who have the most knowledge about the clinical or administrative activities in question. But any number of other individuals wishing to give advice about the educational needs of nursing personnel seem

invariably to enter the picture. These influences are difficult to withstand, particularly when a refusal to accept offerings from other departments in the hospital may be viewed as a lack of interest on the part of the nursing department in working with other departments or in helping to make the services of such departments available to patients. In our zeal to establish good working relations with other departments, we frequently are led to believe that these groups are necessarily capable of determining what nurses need to know. Thus, for example, we may assume that a lecture by the head of central sterilizing on the proper treatment of equipment is an essential part of each nurse's orientation program. It is important to realize that members of other departments will typically tend to look at the nurse's educational needs in terms of their own jobs, the content associated with their own specialties, and the values they hold in relation to their positions. The extent to which their areas of knowledge are appropriate for nurses can be determined only by nurses, if it is true (as we tend to claim) that nursing does have its unique area of expertise. Still other members may doubtless be able to provide nurses with useful information, but decisions about what is needed, who needs it, and when, are ones to be made only by nurses who are capable of assessing nursing care requirements of patients or who understand the processes involved in providing that care. No one individual would be capable of determining all the educational requirements of the nursing staff. The individual in charge of inservice education may well be in the least advantageous position for making such an assessment, except in her own particular area of expertise. She would presumably be able to make gross judgements about such matters as the need for an educational program when a new program of patient care is being instituted. But for the particulars related to that educational need, she would surely have to refer to specialists in the area concerned. The extent of her own involvement might be to recommend that the nurse to be placed in charge of a newly instituted coronary care unit be sent to one of the established programs on coronary care. The experts in such a program would presumably be the ones to determine the educational needs involved.

But even an expert nurse may be distracted from the job of determining educational needs by the assessment of the requirements for patient care in her own area; subtle influences may have even more impact than recommendations from individuals in other departments. A myriad of courses, conferences, movies, film strips, programmed texts, and other resources confront the nurse with such a profusion of material that it may be difficult to make rational decisions about their use. Because of the convenience of preplanned programs, it is a great temptation to build an educational program around them. And there is no doubt that many of these resources can be useful if their selection has been based on a determination that they serve the purposes one has in mind. But this procedure is not always followed. There is a great danger that, rather than the educational needs of a particular department determining the resources to be used, *the availability of the resources suggests the needs*. Such resources are frequently evaluated on their own merits and not on whether they are pertinent to existing educational needs.

Considerations relating to convenience are not the only forces that lead to decisions to use workshops, continuing education programs, and commercially prepared educational materials in the absence of careful assessments of their pertinence to purposes and goals. It is understandable that nurses turn to prepared or predetermined programs for teaching content. Such programs have typically received the seal of approval from outstanding persons in the field, either by virtue of these individuals having themselves developed the materials or programs or by their endorsement of them. Many times one's faith in the quality and relevance of the materials is justified. But because material or a program on a given topic is available does not necessarily mean that it should be incorporated into a given educational program. Frequently it seems to be assumed that exposure to such content can do no harm and *might* yield beneficial results. I suggest that many of our educational efforts are based on just this kind of hope that something good will come from exposure to any content, regardless of its degree of pertinence to the situation at hand.

One frequently finds that when a program is being developed within a department of nursing, the subject matter chosen is selected because it is currently popular. If "patient assessment" is a current faddish topic in nursing circles, the department may decide to provide classes for their staff on the topic, in the absence of a determination that such classes would satisfy any currently existing need. If uncertainty exists about what is required in a particular department in order to provide quality patient care, one may simply choose to make use of whatever activities individuals in other situations deem appropriate. One can derive security from this kind of planning. And if inservice education within a department is evaluated in terms of the extent to which its programs are like those in many hospitals, then a favorable evaluation of them follows as a matter of course.

If patient needs are used as a basis for determining educational needs, however, the decisions can be made only after a careful analysis is conducted (by those having the requisite knowledge) of what the patient needs are and what it will take to satisfy them. The development of a program around a currently popular topic would not be acceptable in the absence of a determination that the topic does in fact have pertinence with respect to existing patient care needs.

It is by no means the case that the solution to an existing problem necessarily lies in the development of an educa-

tional program. The belief that education is the answer for most problems is a common one, particularly when inadequate performance on the part of personnel appears to lie at the heart of the problem. As Mager and Pipe[2] point out, unsatisfactory performance may occur for a variety of reasons. Lack of knowledge is only one of them. Before instituting an educational program, it is important to make certain it is education that is needed. It may be that individuals know what is appropriate, but are not performing adequately for other reasons. Or, it may be that trying to teach a particular behavior would be much less effective than modifying the work situation. There are times when a situational change will result in the introduction of cues that will successfully elicit desired behaviors; in such cases, the investment of time and effort in an educational program might be quite unnecessary and wasteful. The volume by Mager and Pipe is highly recommended to those who are considering the introduction of new educational programs and want to do a careful job of assessing the needs existing within their institutions and of determining how best to meet those needs.

HOW IS THE EDUCATIONAL PROGRAM EVALUATED?

The topic of evaluation will be considered before that of method because the selection of an appropriate method requires prior knowledge of what is to be achieved. If the educator has determined exactly what she wishes to achieve as a result of a teaching program, she is in a position to form clear evaluation criteria and to make intelligent choices both of the content to be covered and the teaching method to be used. Plans for evaluation are crucial in developing a successful educational program. The quality of a program depends heavily on a judicious choice of evaluation criteria. It is my guess that the basis for evaluating most educational offerings is determined after the content and method have been chosen. The student's mastery of the specific content involved is measured, if in fact any evaluation is made. When this practice is followed, one is simply making use of an educational process for its own sake rather than using it as a means of achieving a specified goal that is extrinsic to the process. One of the deficiencies in many of the programmed texts or commercially prepared programs lies in their provisions for evaluation on mastery of the text's contents *per se* rather than on criteria bearing on the use of the content in the work situation. This form of evaluation can differentiate one student's learning from another's, but it will not provide information regarding the effectiveness of *that teaching method or content in producing certain behaviors in the nursing setting*.

There are times when no opportunity exists for observing the ultimate use to be made of information provided in an educational program. This situation is more likely to occur in educational than in practice settings, but even in practice the situation must on occasion be faced. In such cases, it becomes necessary to determine what the student must be able to do at one time (preliminary criterion behavior) so as to be able to perform some specific activity (ultimate criterion behavior) at a later time. For example, the desired future activity of the nurse might include recognizing that a patient is incapable of continuing his nursing care at home and determining what would constitute an appropriate substitute plan that would take into account the constraints and resources in the situation.

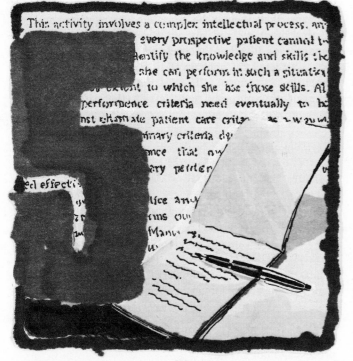

This activity involves a complex intellectual process, and the exact procedure for every prospective patient cannot be taught. But one can identify the knowledge and skills the nurse must have before she can perform in such a situation and evaluate the extent to which she has those skills. All preliminary performance criteria need eventually to be checked against ultimate patient care criteria, as a way of determining if the preliminary criteria do in fact predict the ultimate criteria. But once that relationship has been established, the preliminary performance criteria can be used effectively.

To institute the practice among nurses of establishing evaluation criteria in terms of activities required of the nurse is a difficult job. Many individuals seem to believe that if the specifics of a particular case are not known, one cannot determine in advance what the nurse will be required to do in that case. Some nurses seem to believe that attempts to make predictions in advance result in restrictions on the nurse's ultimate activities and a stifling of her creativity in dealing with patients.

The objectives held by the advocates of either of these beliefs usually pertain to the educational content these individuals deem appropriate, the assumption being that familiarity with such content can be expected to be translated into behaviors providing good patient care. Such individuals may develop mastery of content, but the satisfaction of this objective by no means assures the achievement of quality patient care.

If the fruits of an educational program should take the form of benefits to patients, then it is necessary first to identify what constitutes patient benefits and then to identify those activities the nurse must carry out to achieve them. If the criteria used in the development of educational programs in hospital settings are unrelated to patient care, it is difficult to defend these programs as having pertinence or relevance. It follows that evaluations based on the number of individuals participating or on the opinions of the participants or knowledgeable nurses as to how "good" the program was will not provide assurance that patient care will benefit from the enterprise.

WHAT IS THE BASIS FOR THE CHOICE OF METHOD?

It would be inappropriate to attempt to do any more than touch on the topic of learning methods in the present paper. A good deal is known about "principles of learning," and it certainly behooves individuals responsible for educational programs to be knowledgeable about at least the fundamental ideas involved. However, the danger in becoming preoccupied with such principles is that one may forget the *purpose* of the enterprise. The application of principles of learning and the choice of teaching method must continuously be viewed as means to an end and not as ends in and of themselves.

The *efficiency* of a particular method—in expenditure of time, effort, and money—is a consideration that does not receive proper emphasis in this day of stringent budgetary restrictions and limitations. We tend not to do enough in the way of demanding efficiency in educational programs. We may feel justified in spending $150 for a film which may contain interesting content, but which adds 40 minutes to an educational program without contributing greatly to what is learned and retained by the student and without subtracting in any substantial way from the instructor's investment of time in the program. *The fact that educational material is accurate, interesting, and even generally relevant does not mean it is necessarily appropriate for a given purpose or is the most efficient means of presenting content.*

The director of nursing, the inservice educator, or the supervisor who demands that film strips, movies, programmed instruction texts, lectures, or any other educational material be evaluated with respect to efficiency runs the risk of antagonizing staff members—particularly staff who tend to confuse the entertainment value of a presentation with its effectiveness in the teaching process. There are staff who appear to believe it is useful to provide individuals with all the known information about a topic. But surely certain distinctions need to be made regarding the levels at which different individuals function and the tasks they are responsible for performing. The clinical specialist and the staff nurse should not be expected to benefit comparably from a given body of content. The clinical specialist necessarily studies in depth in order to determine what content is required to provide care needed by patients; such study is part of her job. She does not then expect all staff nurses to acquire all the information she has obtained in order to do their own jobs. For her to provide staff members with content that is not demonstrably necessary for the activities they perform is wasteful. From a utilitarian standpoint, knowledge of "understanding" that is not or cannot be translated into action on the job serves no particular purpose, insofar as hospitals and patients are concerned. (A frequent justification for an educational offering is "to help the nurse understand. . . .") I do not believe one can expect the patient to feel comforted because a staff member has spent a week acquiring knowledge and understanding if this acquisition is not translated into benefits for the patient. Nor should a director of nursing be expected to support an intensive program of study for her supervisory staff, the net result of which is acquisition of information which may be already available in a nursing journal report which presented the pertinent ideas at little expense.

Nursing cannot afford to be casual about the expenditure of time and resources. If we fail to select our educational methods on the basis of considered thought to their effectiveness and to the appropriateness of the content involved (again, judged in terms of the outcomes to be achieved), we are cheating our patients and anyone else who plays a part in financing the hospital's services.

How Are We Doing with Quality Control?

At the risk of belaboring the point, I must repeat that the ultimate test of an educational program is the quality of care given to patients and the ability of staff members to maintain or upgrade that quality. If staff education is viewed as just one factor in the total quality control program, then it must be considered in relation to other existing programs and not as a separate entity. All five standards of JCAH are interrelated. Standard V influences and is affected by implementation of the remaining four standards. The general efficiency of a nursing department in achieving its purposes will reflect the efficiency that characterizes its staff education program.

In examining the preparation of our staff members for providing patient care, we might discover that the supervisor who asks her staff nurses to accompany her when she evaluates patient care has a more effective educational program than does the supervisor who conducts weekly staff development programs. If we decide this is the case, then the former approach can be incorporated as a part of the formal educational program. If we conclude that the weekly meetings comprising the latter approach serve mainly to enhance the morale of the nurses on the staff, then that approach should be recognized for what it is and evaluated accordingly—but not as evidence for adherence to Standard V.

Above all, it must be remembered that education is a process and not an end.

REFERENCES

1. Tosiello, F. University Oriented Inservice Education. *Nurs. Outlook* 12(4):40-41, 1964.
2. Mager, R.F., and Pipe, P. *Analyzing Performance Problems or "You Really Oughta Wanna."* Belmont, Calif.: F. P. Fearon Publishers, Lear Siegler, Inc., Education Division, 1970.

The Case for On-Going Inservice Education

By Betty R. Rudnick and Irma M. Bolte

Betty R. Rudnick obtained her diploma from John Sealy College of Nursing, Galveston, and her B.S. from the University of Houston. Her M.A. and Ed.D. are from Teachers College, Columbia University.

Irma M. Bolte is a graduate, with a diploma in nursing, of St. Mary's Hospital School of Nursing, Quincy, Illinois. Her B.S. in nursing education is from Indiana University and her M.S.N. is from Catholic University of America.

Both authors are in the College of Nursing, University of Kentucky, where Ms. Rudnick is professor of nursing and Ms. Bolte is assistant dean for continuing education and associate professor. This article is reprinted from JONA, March-April, 1971.

Even though the idea of inservice education is far from new, many health-care institutions have either failed to initiate inservice programs or have ineffective programs.

The authors attempt to show the importance of on-going inservice programs, the elements which should be included in such programs and some methods for developing effective programs.

Inservice education is both old and new. It is as old as man's recognition that he could do a better piece of work if he knew more about his job, and as new as the training astronauts undergo to prepare for a trip to the moon. Within the past twenty-five years, health agencies have initiated inservice education programs aimed at developing the nursing staff in order to improve the quality of nursing care. The complexities of the role of nursing team members and the new terminology used in communicating with other health team members have made inservice education an "in thing" for health agencies, particularly hospitals, among other developments.

In spite of this movement of more than two decades, a study of the quality and quantity of inservice education conducted recently in 143 hospitals in the Ohio Valley Region revealed that 13 percent of these hospitals had no formal inservice education program for the nursing employees. Inservice education may be placed in four categories: orientation to the job, skill training, leadership and management development, and on-going education. Those hospitals reporting the existence of inservice education programs indicated that primary emphasis is given to orientation of the new employee and skill training for the nursing assistant. The inclusion of leadership and management development and on-going education in the inservice program was limited and existed for the most part in hospitals with more than 300 beds.[1] While there is an admitted need for inservice education in all four areas, it appears that hospitals in the Ohio Valley Region have just begun to scratch the surface with respect to all areas of inservice education. Unfortunately, this may reflect the national picture.

What is On-Going Education?

On-going education stated simply is this: helping each member of the nursing team work to his highest potential in giving care to the patient.[2] Industry has made on-going education the order of the day and increasingly the responsibility is moving from top management to the supervisory level. Increasingly industries have the attitude that employees must grow on the job or be replaced. Research conducted by several industrial concerns has shown that an employee can do a better job if he has the benefit of a well planned and directed inservice education program.[3]

In addition to the benefits which accrue to the recipients of nursing care from an adequate on-going education program, there are personal benefits received by the members of the nursing team. Attitudes of employees toward the patient, the patient's family and the employee's co-workers are improved. Communications within the nursing team are also improved and the employee's job satisfaction is increased. There is less turnover of employees. The primary advantage of on-going education for nursing personnel is that it keeps the nursing care up to a good standard and updated.

The new graduates from schools of nursing could well be the target for specially planned orientation and on-going inservice education programs. A chronic complaint—justified or not—is that these new graduates come from their programs ill equipped to make the transition from student to worker status. A number of hospitals and agencies plan programs specifically designed to assist the new graduate in learning to apply what she knows in the service setting. This period for the graduate may be likened to the time that the baby kangaroo spends in his mother's pouch between birth and

entry unprotected into the world. A well-planned program for this group may mean the difference between a developing, contributing practitioner of nursing and a frustrated, disillusioned one who may choose to leave nursing altogether or who remains in it and is minimally effective.

Elements of Effective On-Going Education

On-going education, to be effective, must be carefully planned and directed. The study of the 143 hospitals in the Ohio Valley Region showed that 54 percent of the hospitals in one state did not employ a director for inservice education. In these hospitals, when inservice education was offered at all, the director of nursing service assumed responsibility for it.

In many institutions and health agencies which employ inservice education directors, these directors plan and implement centralized programs. Such programs meet the needs of individual personnel and particular patient care units less well than would programs at the level of the patient care unit. When programs are planned on the patient care units, we see this as a responsibility of the head nurse or supervisor.

There are numbers of approaches to developing programs for employees. The first calls for collaboration on the part of hospitals in one geographic area in offering an on-going education program. A select number of employees from each health agency participate and they, in turn, are expected to discuss their experiences with their co-workers and implement as much of their new learnings as feasible. The disadvantage here is that not all employees receive the information at one time and the changes an institution hopes to realize from the on-going education program will not come about as quickly when all personnel are not involved. These programs must be fairly general in nature and cannot deal with skills, information, and situations particular to a single hospital or unit.

The second type of approach is more specific, is confined to one health agency, and

When the program does not meet the needs of the employee, one can expect low interest and poor attendance

involves all levels of personnel. This approach calls for the development of a master plan for on-going education as much as a year ahead. A specific program is planned for each employee level in the nursing department and different times and days are scheduled for each level. There are two disadvantages here: not all personnel can be involved at one time, and personnel are segregated by rank.

A third approach calls for involvement of the supervisor or head nurse in the planning and directing of programs for a specific patient care unit in a health agency. This does not replace a general inservice program of orientation to the total agency or programs to disseminate information and skills necessary for all employees of the agency. The premise of this approach is that a carefully planned and directed program for nursing employees on a specific unit will improve the quality and quantity of care on the unit and increase the job satisfaction of the employee because he gains skills and knowledge which are immediately applicable to the patients he is caring for at that time.

Unfortunately, there is no such thing as an instant or packaged program that will meet the needs of each specific nursing situation. A number of companies do produce programs and equipment designed for hospital inservice education. Most of these are expensive and limited in scope. Comprehensive and specialized programs are still best planned by and for personnel within patient care units. To have a program because it is a fad to have a program is not the goal. When the program does not meet the job needs of the employee, one can expect low interest and poor attendance. The program must help the employee with what he finds most difficult in giving patient care or it will not do anything for his morale. The employee should be involved in the planning. As an involved employee, he takes part in selecting the subjects of the program. The key word here is involvement—it is not only the expressed need of the employee that makes a meaningful program but those needs he is helped to recognize. When the employee understands the purpose of on-going education and

what he needs to do his job effectively, he is ready to make worthwhile suggestions.

Establishing an On-Going Education Program

Most of the foregoing discussion has been in the nature of broad generalities which included the basic elements essential to inservice programs. It is the authors' contention that whether or not an agency is able to employ a director of inservice education, the unit level of on-going education programs is the most important in directly affecting the quality of care and the self-actualization of individual team members. The material that follows is a discussion of some of the practical and realistic features to be dealt with in planning these programs.

Selecting and Planning

The vital core of the unit-level program is its specificity to the needs of the patients and personnel within a unit. If time is made available and space is found and the program then consists of a free film on a general topic or of some speaker who happened to be available, the program is vague and without definition and its value will be lost. Personnel will be dissatisfied and cynical about the value of all programs. Given a group of sick people and a team of nursing personnel, the subject matter for programs is endless. In selecting the subjects for programs, the two major purposes of the programs must be kept in mind. These two major purposes are the improvement of nursing care to the patients and the increased job satisfaction for nursing personnel.

In the beginning the head nurse or supervisor may find the team members floundering in a wide variety of poorly defined ideas for programs. It might be wise for the head nurse or supervisor initially to assess the needs of patients and to select skills or subjects in order of priority. What is most urgently needed for a patient's safety or welfare? What skill or knowledge is most lacking in the personnel? One way of ascertaining this information is the use of the slip technique: each team member is asked to list on a slip of paper the things he needs most to know. When this has been done, a discussion with the staff may indicate the order in which content should be offered; that is, priorities will be established. The needs, as content for the programs, should be expressed in clearly and simply stated goals. Organization of content of the programs which allows time for presentation, for demonstration and for discussion is necessary. It is not enough only to present the material; the head nurse or supervisor must also have some assurance that learning has taken place and some insight into what has been learned. Further, the discussion will reveal, by the questions raised, where weak spots in the program exist and how the program should be modified in the future.

Time

From discussion with large numbers of head nurses and supervisors, it appears that the greatest obstacle to planning and implementing on-going education within a patient care unit is the tight time-frame. This is a realistic problem and not easily solved. It is one that can be dealt with if the head nurse or supervisor is truly committed to the importance of on-going education. Usually we think in terms of hour-long programs. If this is what the personnel on a patient care unit desire, and if an hour is a practical time unit with which to work, there are a number of ways in which to find the hour. Workshifts in hospitals can be arranged so that there is some overlap between the shift coming on and shift going off, and this time can be utilized for programs. Consideration can be given to scheduling part-time personnel to relieve regular staff while they attend programs. A means of seeing that the personnel on the night shift are included is to establish overlap in the morning or to repeat the program during the night. Programs might be taped and one individual on each shift be assigned to comment and answer questions on the taped material. Programs need not be an hour in length to be effective. A format which has been found to be quite effective is the "mini" program: a 15-minute program or series of programs each dealing with a single limited nursing problem.

Space

It is rather sad in the seventies to be still talking about ways for nurses to improvise because their hospitals or health agencies have not considered the continuing education needs of nurses in the first priority of importance. Nevertheless, it is the rule rather than the exception that conference space for nurses on patient care units is either inadequate or unavailable. In many cases such space was not planned in the original design of the unit. In those places where space was planned, it has often been preempted for other purposes. When a quiet spot, free from interruption, has not been provided, what can we do? Our only choice, after making our needs for space known to administration, is the makeshift use of temporarily unoccupied space. Because of the usual noise and activity, the nurses' station is undesirable for this purpose, but it can be used. Any temporary space which does not provide adequate ventilation or seating space and writing area violates teaching-learning tenets and can only be considered as better than nothing. But where motivation is high and programs are interesting, a surprising amount can be accomplished even under undesirable circumstances. A good program in poor space is better than no program at all, and simply having adequate space will not automatically make a program good.

Attendance

There should be a clearly stated policy regarding attendance; this policy should be made known to all employees. Since the purpose of on-going education is the improvement of patient care and since this is the main reason administration would spend time, money, and space on it, even in these permissive times, it is legitimate to require attendance as one criterion for retention and promotion on the job. Keeping in mind the old adage: "you can lead a horse to water but you can't make him drink," we must make the programs pertinent and interesting or we will have only the physical presence of the employees.

On-going education: not entertainment
or a surreptitious nap

Once the programs are of proven benefit to the employees as well as to the patients, an organization might, if it wished, make attendance voluntary or even a privileged opportunity. There will be those who never wish to enforce attendance and perhaps these institutions will meet the greater challenge of making programs so interesting and so relevant to the daily work that the great majority of personnel would wish to attend.

Evaluation

The way you find out if a person has achieved the goals of on-going education is through evaluation. The two most obvious kinds of evaluation are paper-and-pencil tests and observation of performance. In education circles it is held that learning results in changed behavior. The paper-and-pencil test is self-explanatory. In order to know, however, that behavior has been altered for the better, there must be observations made before the program as well as following it. Where the programs have been practical and applicable to patients, it should be simple to observe that one has accomplished his objectives. If there is no observable improvement in patient care, the program was a failure.

Teachers are not made in heaven. Before the head nurse or supervisor can plan, organize, teach, and evaluate, she has to know how. Reality tells us that the majority of head nurses will have had no formal preparation in teaching. Such crucial information about how to teach will make a great deal of difference—not only in the time the head nurse or supervisor must spend in preparing—but also in the final effectiveness of her teaching. There may be formal courses or workshops on how to teach available in the area. If so, the head nurse or supervisor should be encouraged to take advantage of these opportunities. Where no such opportunities exist, there is almost always an individual in the public school system, of even very small communities, who has been educated in teaching methods and who might be called upon to assist the head nurse or supervisor in learning some of the rudiments of planning, teaching, and evaluation.

Summary

A worthwhile on-going education program demands that the supervisor or head nurse use her imagination and that she explore all possibilities to meet the needs of the patient and the nursing staff. The program should be built around the job needs of the staff and should result in growth on the job as well as in improvement of patient care. A wide variety of teaching methods and tools should be used and the supervisor or head nurse should constantly seek the best way to present new information to the employee.

On-going education is not just entertainment or a surreptitious nap while a movie is being shown. The program should be evaluated periodically to determine the impact it has on the patient care unit, and participants should know that evaluations will be made. Just taking a look at the program will not reveal much—it may appear to be lively but, in reality, be dead. The big question to ask is this: Has the program improved patient care? Other questions of lesser importance are: Is it good enough to justify taking the time of the staff? Do the personnel function more effectively as a result of the program? Has it had a positive effect on the staff morale?

If on-going education is to be conducted regularly, it must have the support of the administrative hierarchy. Unless these persons believe in on-going education and recognize the benefits for both the patient and the nursing staff, the program will fail. Rapid changes in the practice of nursing can leave any hospital or health agency behind unless it makes a genuine effort to help the employee *grow on the job*.

REFERENCES

1. OHIO VALLEY REGIONAL MEDICAL PROGRAM. "Regional Survey of Hospital Inservice Programs." 1969. (unpublished OVRMP report)
2. McPHETRIDGE, MAE. "On-Going Inservice Education." Paper presented at Management for Nursing Care Conference, University of Kentucky College of Nursing, Lexington, Kentucky, March, 1969.
3. PAUL, WILLIAM J. JR., ROBERTSON, KEITH B., and HERZBERG, FREDERICK. "Job Enrichment Pays Off." *Harvard Business Review*, 47:61-71, March, April 1969.

NO ONE SET OF RULES APPLIES

by **MARJORIE MOORE CANTOR**

Marjorie Moore Cantor is also the author of the second article in this reader and her biographic data appears there. This article is reprinted from JONA, November-December, 1973.

In my capacity as Associate Director for Staff Development at the University of Iowa Hospitals and Clinics, I frequently receive letters from other nursing departments seeking information about our staff development program. Although happy to provide the information requested, I typically feel uneasy about answering these requests because of the difficulties encountered in describing the complex structure and particular conditions that characterize our educational program. Like any other program within a department of nursing, a staff development program is inextricably connected with virtually all other existing programs and it reflects the department's philosophy of nursing, style of administration, beliefs about the educational process, and the resources available to it.

An additional source of concern to me is that a given staff development program will work well in one institution and be totally inappropriate in another.

Although the ostensible goal of all staff development programs is the preparation of staff to provide quality patient care, and standards set up by the various accrediting agencies provide apparently applicable guidelines, it does not follow that staff development programs are, or necessarily should be, similar to one another. The methods and procedures adopted in following guidelines and achieving goals differ considerably across programs. Such variability seems virtually inevitable, given the differences in program philosophies, structures, and resources, not to mention the individual personalities involved.

Available descriptions of inservice education programs seldom include information about the conditions necessary for the functioning of the program. Neither do they disclose the extent to which the methods employed have been evaluated for efficiency and effectiveness, or the philosophy of nursing or education that underlies the program. To duplicate a given program in another setting could prove both costly and unrewarding. For example, it is possible that an impressive offering in a particular setting, using the most carefully evaluated advanced teaching methods, carefully evaluated for effectiveness, will be excessively costly in terms of the benefits derived from it. Further, it is not unusual for educational programs to be set up by means of techniques and materials that do indeed achieve the intended results, but with a failure to recognize that the same results might have been achieved at much less cost or with much less effort. Given a restricted educational budget, a nursing department will hardly benefit from trying to duplicate programs functioning successfully in more amply endowed settings.

Recommendations from accrediting agencies and leaders in the field can provide ammunition for a director of nursing when she is arguing for the adoption of certain educational programs, and hence for the investment necessary to implement them. But there are limits beyond which an agency cannot go. Considering the many programs within the agency competing for funds, one can hardly expect an endless supply of money to be allocated for strictly educational purposes.

Departments that have abundant resources may deliberately choose not to use their money for bigger and "better" educational programs. The development of programs of care for specific groups of patients, with emphasis on evaluating the nursing techniques involved, might be regarded as more in keeping with the department's philosophy of nursing and staff development than would be the acquisition of prepared materials for use in a new or expanded educational program. Such a judgment would be particularly appropriate if the individuals in responsible positions in such a department were concerned about the quality of available educational materials but did not feel equipped to make discriminating choices or had no interest in investing the time and effort needed to do so.

In contrast, an equally well endowed department might choose to invest extensively in educational materials with a view toward evaluating them and subsequently using the best of them. In view of the skills and interests required to engage effectively in this project, such an investment of resources could be highly appropriate and productive. In any case, the wisest investment will be made by those who have analyzed their settings and philosophies to determine the approach that is most appropriate for them.

Many factors determine the extent to which a given model for staff education will provide an effective means of preparing staff members. Numerous models and methods of approach also exist. Perhaps the frustrations experienced by some inservice training personnel arise from their attempts to fit inappropriate models to their settings, not having recognized that the conditions necessary for the effective use of the chosen models are not present in their situations.

Staff development is an important aspect of the total program of nursing care. It can play a crucial role in determining the quality of care given. But if it is to be effective in this regard, it must be planned in relation to all other existing programs in the department. Staffing programs, performance evaluation and quality control programs, and administrative operations all relate importantly to staff education concerns. Staff development personnel who lack constant input about these programs are not likely to meet the educational needs of the nursing staff.

When a staff development program is being established or remodeled, certain basic decisions must be made. Those in charge must give considerable thought to making choices that are consistent with the total program of care or the decisions will be made by default because those individuals who should shoulder the responsibility fail to do so. Obviously, the former approach is preferable and necessitates an examination on the part of the director of nursing, her designate, or both, of the total operation. Special emphasis should be given to the objectives of the program in order to determine: (1) where decisions about content for staff development activities shall reside; (2) what shall be the scope of, the placement of, and the priorities given to, the various offerings; (3) where the accountability for the results of the educational program shall reside; (4) what methods of evaluation will be used; (5) what the method and amount of funding will be; (6) what qualifications will be required of the individuals belonging to the staff development unit; and (7) how resources and experts will be identified and used. I believe these issues are of crucial importance when one is planning a staff development program. Consequently, they are the topics to which subsequent columns in this series will be devoted. A few preliminary observations regarding them follow in the remainder of this introductory column.

Decision making and accountability regarding needed educational programs for their results should take into account the philosophies of staff members concerning nursing practice and administration. Preferences in styles of practice should be taken into account, as should the skills of individuals working at the various levels of authority within the department. Even if one believes that the expert practitioner should be responsible for identifying the requisite skills, it may nonetheless be the case that the specialists on hand may not, despite their expertise in practice, be able to identify program requirements perceptively. In such a case, the director might appropriately choose to retain the identification function until her staff acquires the knowledge needed to engage effectively in this process.

If the director of nursing has an administrative style that requires extensive staff involvement in decision making, she might conclude that the prerogative for making staff development decisions would be out of harmony with her general mode of functioning. An analysis of priorities and, particularly, long-term goals will likely be useful in helping her decide the appropriate stance to take on this issue.

The beliefs about nursing and nursing education held by the physicians and administrators in the general setting will certainly influence the kind of funding that can be expected, as well as the amount and kind of encouragement that will be provided any programs that are implemented. What the nursing department has already accomplished in preparation of staff will doubtless influence the thinking of such individuals. But at some point, the nursing director undoubtedly will find that progress (or the lack of it) will depend very heavily on the attitudes held by physicians and administrators. Failure to recognize the existence of such attitudes would prevent the director from considering ways of accommodating these attitudes to the best advantage of her department.

The type and size of staff presently functioning in the department will certainly have a bearing on the kind of staff development program that will be needed and that can be implemented. A nursing department in which new staff must be moved very quickly into positions of responsibility must approach the educational process with a set of premises different from those of a department in which there exists overlap time or a high staffing rate.

If new personnel are to be hired to participate in a staff development program, the issue of qualifications for the positions in question arises. Realistically, one must take into account who is available for such positions, how much can be afforded in salaries, and in what areas the greatest need for expertise exists. Reciprocally, those available for hire at the salaries that can be afforded will, to a considerable extent, determine the kind of program that can be developed.

It is frequently said that one should not rely on physicians for the education of nurses. But if the physician is the only person available having the requisite information about patient care requirements, it may be necessary to depend on him for staff education, at least until nursing personnel gain the necessary knowledge. Under such circumstances, it is important to take steps to insure that the basic control of nursing not be surrendered to others in the process.

Staff development programs can develop like Topsy. They can also be *designed* to make the most of what is available in order to provide the best fit within the total departmental operation. Perhaps the most important consideration involves the understanding that even when one's goal is directed to the provision of quality patient care, various ways of achieving that goal exist. In my opinion, too much concern has been expressed about whether or not staff development programs conform to set patterns and not enough concern about whether or not the department is making the most effective and efficient use of the available resources for the benefit of the patient. Many unsupported assumptions regarding staff education become reiterated, frequently being treated as if they are of divine origin. Certain practices are implemented even when there is evidence to indicate that they are not effective for the purpose at hand. It is my hope that by examining some of the relevant issues in subsequent columns in this series, we can establish meaningful premises on which to develop realistic staff education programs.

Who Decides and Who is Accountable

This is the third article by **Marjorie Moore Cantor** appearing in this reader. Her biographic data appears with the first article. This article is reprinted from JONA, May-June, 1974.

If it can be assumed that staff education plays an integral role in preparing staff members to provide high quality nursing care, then the questions of who should make major decisions about educational programs and how the decisions should be made take on considerable importance. In practice, it seems that much of the planning for staff development occurs independently of planning focused on quality patient care. Frequently, decisions about educational content, about the amounts of emphasis to be placed on specific programs, and about cost allocations are made by persons having no responsibility for the quality of care to be provided. Or, when decisions are made by those responsible for the quality of care to be provided, it is not necessarily the case that such persons are able to determine what is required to prepare the staff to maintain a certain quality of care.

Obviously the director of nursing bears the ultimate responsibility for her department's educational program, as she does for all other aspects of her unit's functioning. But only in the smallest of hospitals can the director of nursing make all the decisions about staff preparation, assure that the ongoing goals of the educational program are commensurate with those of the nursing department in general, and make certain that the content acquired in the educational program is applied in the practice of nursing within the clinical setting. In the majority of situations, these functions must be delegated to others. But since the quality of care that patients receive is directly related to the knowledge and skill of the individuals providing that care, the delegation of the responsibility for making decisions about the staff development program is not a step to be taken lightly. Of course, the director of nursing cannot by delegation of the responsibility divest herself of accountability for the quality of the decisions made and for the effectiveness of the program provided the staff. It is extremely important that she both recognize and take seriously the existence of a relationship between educational programs and accountability for quality of care.

The patient who develops a complication because the nurse failed to recognize the importance of certain symptoms will hardly be comforted by the knowledge that the nursing department had an excellent orientation program, but that those exposed to it failed to see the relevance of the program's content to their day-by-day nursing practice. Given the application of rigorous evaluation techniques to their staff development programs, it might surprise many directors of nursing to discover how frequently their inservice programs are developed around content instead of nursing care or performance objectives and how often performance criteria, when they are designated as desirable and necessary, are not applied within the clinical setting.

Even the director of nursing who believes she has kept a close eye on her department's staff education programs and who takes an active role in decisions about staff preparation might find that decisions about program content and focus have been taken over by individuals whose standards differ from hers or whose goals are not consistent with those of the nursing department. The hospital culture and the nature of the nursing profession tend to encourage individuals to accept practices without examining them for effectiveness or even for their purposes. Therefore a director of nursing might well be unaware of the discrepancies existing between what is thought to be happening and what is actually the case. Indications that should serve as warnings exist within a department when personnel fail to recognize the staff development function as essential to the guarantee of quality care to patients and when all staff members are not committed to the same standards of performance.

Not uncommonly, "selling" the staff development program to personnel constitutes a central focus of concern in its operation; the chances are good in such cases that those implementing the nursing care programs fail to see a relationship between the existing educational offerings and what they perceive as a desirable staff preparation. Sometimes general agreement exists about the appropriateness of the educational content being provided, but the individuals for whom the classes are intended, or their supervisors, repeatedly justify absences from those classes. It would appear here that attendance is being seen as the educational program's goal rather than as a means of obtaining information needed for the betterment of patient care. If the supervisors do not insist that staff members attend the classes or that classes be scheduled in order to make attendance possible, then they are either failing to maintain the standards toward which the class content is oriented or they believe the classes are not pertinent to what they view as being desirable departmental standards. It is possible that certain offerings are made available to staff for their own self-improvement, with attendance being a matter of choice for them. Whether the sessions are deemed necessary for the achievement of quality nursing care or simply as an activity designed for the benefit of the individual staff member, the question of motivation should hardly arise if the educational program is successfully serving the purpose for which it is intended.

If decisions about what to include in continuing inservice education or orientation programs are made by asking new staff members what they need, or by a staff member who is having a "learning experience" as chairman of an inservice continuing education committee, or by a vote of the supervisors, or by physicians, hospital administrators, or inservice education coordinators, then the standard for staff preparation are being established by individuals who are not accountable for the performance of the staff. Although the new employee might seem to be an appropriate individual to indicate what she needs, she is in fact likely to be least qualified to provide this information. It is difficult to see how an individual in need of certain content can make appropriate judgments about what that content ought to be. The new employee can indicate what she herself is concerned about and what she sees as constituting her needs at the moment. But it is unreasonable to expect her to be able to indicate what she needs in order to meet the department's objectives.

Having the staff nurse set up continuing education programs for the service or de-partment might be a way to build her morale, but such an approach would also serve to reinforce the idea that inservice education is designed for interest or entertainment value rather than to facilitate the meeting of standards of care. Similarly, permitting supervisors to vote might seem to be a way of meeting their needs, but they may lack a thorough understanding of their own particular problems of nursing care delivery; or they may have such an understanding but might feel compelled to settle for something they think would be palatable to all the staff members concerned, including those whose standards differ from theirs.

The hospital administrator may be accountable for the care his hospital's nurses provide, but he lacks the requisite nursing knowledge regarding what constitutes acceptable or preferred performance. The inservice education coordinator, even if she is a nurse, does not have to answer for the quality of the care provided patients. The physician might seem to be an appropriate individual to make decisions about staff education; it is certainly the case that he can be an extremely useful source of information about the care requirements of the patients. But it must be remembered that he tends to be insular in his perception of patient care problems. He tends to set priorities on his own terms and may have few compunctions about using nursing department funds to enhance his clinical area at the expense of some other ones in the hospital. It is well to keep in mind that the medical director of the coronary care unit does not have to answer for a lack of prepared staff to care for a patient having hip replacement surgery on orthopedics.

If an individual's recommendations about staff education needs are accepted simply because he or she is an "expert"—whether a physician, a nursing supervisor, a clinical nursing specialist, or a nursing college professor—there is great danger that the emphasis is being placed on knowledge per se rather than on the results to be achieved with patients. Unless such individuals are required to document the existence of the need and the objectives that can be expected to be achieved as a result of the recommended experience, the director of nursing has no basis on which to determine whether a given educational offering merits the allocation of time, money, and effort more than does any other offering or activity.

If a schism exists between the staff development group and the service personnel—if either group chronically complains about what the other is doing—it is highly likely that the two groups are not viewing the purposes and objectives of the staff development program in the same way. Obviously, one can expect certain disagreements to arise, but such disputes should be concerned with resolving specific problems; they should not permeate the ongoing relationships between the two groups. If neither dissension nor cooperative involvement is present, the standards for staff performance and the philosophy supposedly held by the department may not be clear enough to give direction to either group. If the department does not have clear standards of performance or a firm commitment to standards, the various facets of the staff development program will likely be based on several standards and will involve varying levels of quality. If the staff development group is setting up programs that compel unilateral adjustments on the part of service personnel without any input from such personnel, it is likely that the service people will be unsympathetic with the programs and the standards they espouse. On the other hand, if the staff development personnel are expected to develop programs in the absence of information about other existing programs within the department, or if they are trying to adapt to staffing patterns, to the introduction of new programs of care, or to changes in philosophy of care without knowledge of the plans or changes involved, it can hardly be expected that they will be able to organize and maintain an effective instructional program.

Since the director of nursing cannot herself directly plan, implement, and evaluate the results of the staff development program, she needs to have some basis on which to decide how she should delegate functions associated with staff education. To be qualified to make decisions about staff education, one needs to be knowledgeable about: (1) the job requirements involved; (2) the content required by the individuals who will perform the activities; and (3) the method of presentation that will maximize the likelihood of efficient, effective acquisition and long-term retention of the content. It is unlikely that all this knowledge will be possessed by any one individual per service. In addition, the most efficient use of talent may not be entailed if one or more individuals responsible for delivering the service to patients are asked to do all the teaching involved. The individual who actually presents a given segment of content might not be held accountable for the performance of duties related to that content in the clinical setting. But it is essential that the same standards of performance be held by both the individual who is accountable (e.g., the nursing supervisor) and the person who does the teaching. This common committment can be achieved only if nursing performance standards are made explicit, are endorsed by the nursing administrative

staff, and are applied to the performance of all staff members, and only if the educational programs are considered successful to the extent that they are directed to and result in the achievement of those goals. The question of who should determine the content to be included in such programs is not so much at issue as is the question of the basis on which such decisions are made and the relevance of the educational offering to stated patient care objectives. Ideally, the one whom the director of nursing holds accountable for care should be the individual who knows what skills and knowledge are required—i.e., the supervisor or head nurse. Unfortunately, such an individual may have difficulty relating the educational preparation problem to the problem of providing quality patient care. This does not mean that this individual fails to provide quality care—the care she and her staff provide may be excellent. But she may be unable to formulate a precise statement of the specific preparatory activities required to achieve a given result. Establishing priorities regarding the content to be learned might prove an even more difficult task if the individual in question has been accustomed to think about the educational process along traditional nursing school lines. The traditional approach does not in general appear to have placed much emphasis on the formulation of educational priorities based on *patient care* priorities. Rather, the focus has predominantly been on nursing content and the nursing process itself, more or less divorced from considerations pertaining directly to patient care outcomes.

It is possible that the practicing nurse who seems to be unable to bridge the gap between nursing practice and educational preparation has this apparent deficit mainly because the activity has never been demanded of her. The director of nursing probably cannot specify the performances necessary for the achievement of given nursing outcomes, but she can establish the expectation that staff education programs will be developed on the basis of explicit performance objectives directly concerned with meeting patient care criteria. This expectation would appropriately apply to the contributions made by both the practitioners and any individuals in the department whose sole or major responsibility is the development of inservice education programs. The director should expect all of these individuals to be able to demonstrate the relationship between recommended teaching methods and content, on the one hand, and the achievement of specified performance objectives on the other. Finally, while she probably must depend on these various individuals to formulate *specific* standards and patient care objectives, she should have some explicitly stated *general* standards in mind,

standards that are clearly focused on excellence and on quality patient care.

The effectiveness of the staff development program is a responsibility of the director of nursing. She needs to be certain that the program results in appropriately prepared staff. This she can do in part by setting up criteria that specify what is needed for a successful educational program. These criteria might well include the following:

1. Every clinical service or unit should have a functioning system for certifying that a new employee is capable of assuming the responsibilities associated with each aspect of her job before she is expected to take on those responsibilities. Those activities most crucial to the patient's welfare should come earliest in the training sequence.

2. The individuals responsible for the educational programs should demonstrate the use of the certification procedures employed in the systems mentioned above as a means of specifying the objectives of orientation and inservice education programs. The most effective and efficient methods of presentation should be used to maximize the probabilities of eliciting the desired behaviors when they are needed.

3. Individuals responsible for service areas should make periodic reports about staff education needs, based on a study of problems encountered in maintaining patient care standards.

4. Continuing education programs should be directed toward the achievement of stated objectives of performance, these being based on the results to be achieved with patients.

5. The objectives of existing continuing education programs, formulated on a department-wide basis, should be established as standards of performance on the various clinical areas and incorporated into the performance evaluation systems of those areas.

A department that fulfills these criteria would be one in which decisions regarding staff development would be based on knowledge about what is needed to achieve quality patient care and in which staff members would be commited to the idea of certified staff preparation.

As a postscript, it should perhaps be noted that a department might well develop and maintain staff development activities for reasons not directly related to practice within the clinical settings. Provision of experiences for the general benefit of the staff might be part of a continuing education program within an institution. The important point to remember is that these kinds of activities should be viewed as additions to the staff development program and not as substitutes for activities that maintain or enhance the quality of patient care.

Continuing Education Climatology

By Jean E. Schweer

Jean E. Schweer received her R.N. from the Memorial Hospital School of Nursing in South Bend, Indiana. She earned a B.S. in nursing education with a major in teaching medical-surgical nursing and an M.S. in nursing education with a major in administration in schools of nursing at Indiana University School of Education.

In addition, Miss Schweer has participated in doctoral study in adult education at Indiana University. She is presently professor of nursing and director of continuing education, Indiana University School of Nursing. This article is reprinted from JONA, January-February, 1971.

The proliferation of continuing education programs demonstrates the need for in-service education. The programs generally suffer from lack of acceptance as a major endeavor requiring a high priority. Developing a working environment conducive to continual learning requires nursing administrators to serve as role-models. They must provide a climate that allows learners the freedom to determine their learning needs and to implement change through application of newly learned skills and knowledge.

Continuing education courses should consider the eight concerns identified as basic factors in providing a climate for fostering a concept of continuing education that is rewarding to all levels of personnel.

Hospitals, public health agencies, and other types of health facilities, caught up in the rapid growth of scientific knowledge and technological advances, are struggling to deliver the kinds of health care required by our rapidly growing population. Nurses now have unlimited opportunities to enhance their professional stature by assuming the initiative for providing preventive and therapeutic health care in a variety of new approaches and physical settings.

The resulting rapid and sporadic growth of various kinds of highly specialized nursing care often leads to educational crash programs designed to teach a series of highly technical skills to a select group of nurses in a particular setting. The object is to provide safe, therapeutic care to patients who are, in fact, being admitted for this highly specialized care *before*

adequate opportunities for learning have been provided for the staff.

Nurses all too often fail to recognize the related need for planned, continued learning as a part of their lifelong commitment to nursing practice. A most familiar response of nurses is that their day-to-day, on-the-job learning opportunities are quite sufficient for providing them with the knowledge and skills they need to be effective practitioners.

The learning climate must be supportive if professional nurses are to develop this concept of learning as a lifelong activity. Schools of nursing can create a desirable climate by administrative support of continued learning and by making opportunities available to faculty for the additional learning experiences they need to keep up with changing practice. Faculty members must serve as role models and assume responsibility for their own continuous self-improvement, and must integrate the concept of continuing education into various aspects of the curriculum. Students will then accept continuous learning as a natural part of their professional responsibility.

Of even greater significance in developing this concept of continuing education is the climate maintained by the clinical setting, whether hospital, public health agency, or another kind of health facility in which nurses function, whether as students or as professional practitioners. The climate for learning in the work situation is set by top administrative personnel and filters through to supervisory and staff levels. Therefore, nursing administrators must serve as role-models in developing and maintaining a working environment that is conducive to continual learning. They must be interested not only in systematic, planned education programs, but in learning from colleagues and other personnel, both at the administrative and clinical levels. Belief in the concept of continuing education must be reflected by clinical practice that allows personnel to pool their resources while using problem solving approaches to patient care to test their ideas or to seek further knowledge and skills. One cannot overemphasize the importance of the administrator's commitment to provide opportunities for nurses to seek further educational experiences.

Nurses must also have the freedom to test or apply significant new knowledge in their work situations. Their total commitment to continued learning can be achieved only if the learners are given freedom to: (1) make their own decisions about participating in a course, (2) determine their own objectives for learning, and (3) implement changes in the work situation based on application of new knowledge and skills. All too often we encounter course participants who express hostility about having been sent to a course without any desire to attend, •or indeed without any knowledge of the course other than that attendance is required. A greater evil often encountered even by those who were required to attend is a lack of administrative support when they return to the job highly motivated to make changes based on the knowledge and skills gained from the experience.

Continuing education is a two-dimensional process: (1) participation in systematic, planned courses offered by institutions of higher education through intensive, non-credit courses, or courses leading to an advanced degree; and (2) individual growth through independent study and development of strategic judgments regarding priorities which will contribute to top-level nursing performance.

Although the concept of continuing education is not new to other educational and professional fields, its acceptance by the nursing profession has been much slower. Many good programs are, however, already operational and many emerging programs are offering well planned, clinically oriented courses taught by authorities. In contrast to those who view the future of continuing education in nursing with a bit of skepticism, Malcolm Knowles predicts, in a thought-provoking statement, that society will come to consider continuing education as much a necessity for satisfying living as is the education of children today.

If we subscribe to the theory that the individual is responsible for a lifetime of learning, whose responsibility is it to foster the development of this kind of commitment as part of professional practice? One cannot discount the valuable learning opportunities that are present in day-to-day nursing practice, but unfortunately this kind of learning is incidental and seldom available when it is needed by all personnel. In recognition of this, hospitals, agencies, and schools have attempted to provide in-service education programs of varying kinds. Some of these have developed into highly sophisticated teaching departments, some have merely provided information essential to practice in a specific area of a given institution, some have provided monthly meetings designed to meet the needs of the institution rather than the needs of the participants. All have doubtless met at least minimal needs, but the ultimate value for improvement of patient care can be seriously questioned.

As an administrator, I do not have to remind you about the rapidity of growth or change you are experiencing. These changes, coupled with the growing complexity of the world, make it imperative that educational institutions and health agencies accept the responsibility for continued learning, albeit with a different focus. Health agencies and institutions have the responsibility to provide excellent health care for the consumer. There are unlimited opportunities to teach that which is needed to uphold the goal of excellence in health care delivery, but the most important question is: who teaches the teachers in these institutions and agencies?

The crux of the matter is that we must provide continuing education courses which allow for active learner participation and have relevance readily apparent to the learner. The American Nurses' Association has supported the idea that institutions of higher education should assume responsibility for continuing education so that learners can benefit from programs that are educationally sound and taught by experts. Colleges and universities genuinely committed to continuing education are concerned first about the needs of the learners and the environment in which they function, and second, the

The individual is responsible for a
lifetime of learning

pragmatic development of the program in tune with these needs. Those of us in continuing education programs in universities, can be guided by the enthusiastic response and feedback from learners who attend these courses. Beyond the multitude of problems relating to the mechanics of staffing, financing, and scheduling, I think I can speak for many of my counterparts about some of our concerns for the future programming of continuing education courses:

1) Administrators of service agencies and schools of nursing must place great enough value on the ultimate results of continuing education programs to accept the responsibility for: providing opportunities for personnel to attend courses away from their own work situation; assuming some financial support for sending personnel to courses; providing universities with measurable feedback about the results of the courses in terms of improved patient services; and offering suggestions and qualified personnel for the planning and presentation of courses. Those who have a positive commitment to continuing education are seeking out those agencies and institutions having a similar commitment and who do, in fact, provide a favorable climate for learning for their personnel.

2) Continuing education courses should be planned so that a "spread effect" can be achieved, wherever possible. Quality courses in continuing education often have enrollments limited to give the participants ample opportunity to take part in actual learning activities. It should be possible for most of this nucleus of participants to return to their own communities and conduct similar programs for other nurses and non-professional nursing personnel.

3) For the most part, colleges and universities are reluctant to offer continuing nursing education courses for personnel other than professional nurses unless a team approach is used, because of the differences in the objectives for teaching each level of personnel. Even though we recognize the need for continuing education for all levels, we feel committed to provide first for high quality continuing education programs for professional nurses. Administrative personnel can accomplish the "spread effect" by recruiting appropriate personnel to attend continuing education courses for the purpose of returning to

their own institutions to teach non-professional personnel and/or other professional nurses in the local area.

4) The rapidly changing health care patterns, the need for increased numbers of personnel, and the proliferation of new technological tools suggests that universities, hospitals, community agencies, and educational technology centers need to pool their unique contributions in cooperative programs reaching professional nurses throughout large geographical areas. In addition to cost savings, such cooperative efforts would avoid duplication of services. The total program would be enriched because of the unique contributions each institution would make, which would otherwise be confined to a small group. As a result many people at the local level will become involved in helping to plan programs as well as in the learning activities.

5) Those responsible for planning and teaching in the area of continuing education must be always mindful that they are dealing with adult learners who have specific needs, both professional and personal, that must be taken into account when planning, presenting, and evaluating programs. Emphasis should be on a process design for program development that produces the content needed to best meet the needs of the adult learners. Malcolm Knowles describes this kind of an approach in greater depth, using a new term, "the adragogical approach". His discussion bears careful consideration for those committed to meeting the needs of adults in the 1970's.

6) The expense of taking a high quality continuing education course should not be a factor for professional nurses. Administrators must share the responsibility for helping their personnel recognize the value of education, regardless of the cost, and should make economic assistance available as part of their fringe benefit program. This is one of the few fringe benefits that really "pays off" for both the employer and the employee in ultimate improvement in health care. Administrators must look at the total effect such programs have on patient care. The initial investment may appear dubious because of rapid personnel turnover, but patients somewhere else may benefit from the increased knowledge and skill of the

nurse. Furthermore, one nurse lost may be replaced by one who has had the benefit of a similar education program elsewhere.

7) Professional nurses need to show more concern about the value of their learning activities relating to the delivery of health care, job satisfaction, and self-growth.

8) The overwhelming need of learners to receive credits or grades as external rewards for time, effort, and money spent in taking a course indicates a lack of maturity. Educators and administrators must change such behavior, either during students' basic educational experiences or during subsequent work experiences.

Graduates of today's nursing programs and nurses returning to practice need assistance, support, and encouragement from those in administrative positions. These factors as discussed here furnish the climate, either a positive or a negative one, for continuing education. Perhaps they can serve as a checklist to help you build a continuing education climate that is satisfying to you, to your personnel, and ultimately to your patients.

BIBLIOGRAPHY

AMERICAN NURSES ASSOCIATION. "Avenues for Continued Learning." New York, American Nurses Association, 1967.

SIMMS, LAURA L. "The Role of the Practitioner in Continuing Education." *Continuing Education for Nursing/Tools and Techniques.* New York, American Nurses Association, 1968, pp. 6-7.

COOPER, SIGNE S. "Continuing Education: An Imperative for Nurses." *Nursing Forum* 7:289-297, 1968.

POPIEL, ELDA S. "The Many Facets of Continuing Education in Nursing." *Journal of Nursing Education* 8:3-13, Jan. 1969.

KNOWLES, MALCOLM S. "Gearing Adult Education for the Seventies." *Journal of Continuing Education in Nursing* 1:11, May 1970.

Ibid, pp. 14-16.

Setting the Stage for Teaching Ancillary Personnel

Joan C. Murphy

"Where are you now?" is a pointed and common question used by young people today to keep "in tune" with one another after a passage of time or events. It means how are you at this moment in life as regards your whole being. The ability to relate, which is implied in this phrase, is really the secret of effectiveness in training ancillary health personnel. It is not what you teach or how you teach it that matters. It is how you "set the stage" for teaching that is important and influences heavily the nature of your continuing educational relationship.

On the first day in training, Mr. or Mrs. X present their entire being, not just a reasonable ability to learn and act within some predetermined format. We seldom know, at first, what brings a new employee to this setting, but most experienced instructors agree that there usually is an inner desire to help, to give of themselves.

It is to the advantage of the employee, patient, and institution to capitalize on the inner beauty which motivates people to work in health agencies. To capitalize requires a high degree of understanding; little acts become very important. You want your new employee to quickly realize that you are open to him as an equal, completely receptive and anxious to know his potentials and his desires, as well as eager to assist him in whatever way possible. This response is not always easily attainable. Amongst other responses, the instructor must exert real effort to know herself and how she is seen by others.

In orienting and training new ancillary personnel a multi-dimensional approach must be used if these processes are to have a lasting effect. We must learn to reach out to our colleagues and subordinates, i.e., tune into their "wave-lengths." Hopefully we do this with patients, but we forget that employees are people too! Acceptance of employees with a "tuned in" attitude should reinforce the probability that patients will be accepted with the same openness.

On the first encounter the instructor should warmly welcome the new employee with a handshake, warm smile, and an introduction. It must be real, not the perfunctory kind often seen in business. I recall an instance when this initial introduction was all a particular woman could manage on her first day. A recent widow, it required great psychological energy to leave her home after years of being there and return to work. She was literally exhausted by nine A.M.! Given acceptance and understanding, she went home and returned the next day for orientation. Time has proved her a satisfied and valuable employee!

Realistically the time available for initial training of employees is limited. Time spent in establishing a proper climate is a good investment, however. First, and probably most important, begin the first day getting to know each other—employer and employee—by verbalizing about the job. Traditionally the employee is overwhelmed by the objective facts about the institution, personnel policies, and the like. Meanwhile, 50 percent of their thoughts may be centered on the new babysitter at home, 10 percent on how to get home, 25 percent on being hungry, 10 percent on needing to go to the lavatory, and only 5 percent on what is being said. But if you "tune in" initially to what's on everyone's mind, you gain their full attention because you are "with them."

The next step is to initiate conversation on key areas regarding the aging process; normal growth and development and, especially, how it coincides with illness and wellness. This type of conversation is especially effective in

---

Joan Murphy received a B.S. degree in nursing from Nazareth College in Rochester, New York. In addition to teaching ancillary personnel, Miss Murphy has spent much of her professional interest in better care for our elderly. This article is reprinted from JONA, November-December, 1971.

the nursing home setting. Almost universally the topic of death will come up at this time and, often, deep feelings emerge. Especially relevant are feelings about recent deaths of relatives, for these feelings have a potential for helping or hindering patient care and should be handled accordingly. Talking openly on such topics as death, grieving, separation, and the meaning of life automatically draws the class together in a strong bond.

Throughout the actual lessons it is extremely valuable to include personal patient care experiences, not only examples of technical care and the patient reactions, but examples of real person to person encounter on the patient care level. This latter method sparks enthusiasm in the employee who desires to reach out on a human level. It evokes a psychological reaction in the class and also gives them a picture of staff-patient rapport before they go to the units.

Perhaps the reader will question this emphasis on building rapport among ancillary personnel at the orientation phase. There are many reasons for this emphasis, but primarily it is because the ancillary personnel work with and relate to the patient. Professionals, despite their desire to return to the bedside, seem to have difficulty getting there free enough to relate as whole persons. Whatever the restraint, paperwork, pills, paraprofessional relationships, or the "professional taboo" on chatting with patients, professionals are there in spirit only.

The emphasis on building rapport with the ancillary employees arises from the fact that they are available to genuinely relate to the whole patient. Usually the ancillary employee understands at least as much about the patient's illness as does the patient, but generally does not bear as much responsibility for this "ill" segment as does the professional. This leaves the ancillary employee free, as a part of the health team, to focus on the "healthy" segments of the patient's being, by behaviors such as the following.

1. *Chatting with the patient,* during or apart from giving care, on such topics as family, children, work, cultural events, television programs, sports, and the like.

2. *Conducting remotivation sessions* with groups of eight to ten patients (after given sufficient training to do so).

3. *Assisting the professional* in conducting group therapy sessions.

4. *Encouraging the patients* to form "reading groups."

Focusing on the healthy segments of a patients being is a beginning toward recognizing our responsibility for the whole being, and the ancillary staff can play a very significant role in that recognition! The focus on illness is but a minute segment of total health care, and encouraging ancillary health personnel to build on the positive makes them a vital part of the health team.

Setting the stage properly has many advantages:

1. The employee senses *personal interest* on the part of the instructor.

2. Ego support provokes *attention* on the part of the learner.

3. The *person centeredness* hopefully will be carried to the patient.

4. There will be a realization of our *responsibility* toward the well aspects of the individual as well as toward his illness state.

5. *Job satisfaction* is promoted.

Setting the stage for instruction is only the beginning, of course, in a long learning relationship, but so very important. Having read this brief article, are you now going to ask yourself where you are at?

Lighting the Candle— An Experiment in Cooperative Continuing Education

By Elida L. Mundt

This is a report of an experiment in faculty development by four hospital schools of nursing. The author describes the objectives and rationale for a joint program of continuing education and events leading to its approval as a federal project grant sponsored by the Department of Health, Education and Welfare.

Problems of organization, budget, and implementation are explored. Growth of individual faculty members is highlighted and evaluation results suggest the value of this experiment as a pattern for others, not only for other faculty groups but also for nursing service staff of hospitals and similar health agencies.

Background and Rationale

Any educational institution must provide a sufficient number of adequately qualified faculty members to instruct, guide, and supervise students.[1] Few nursing administrators would quarrel with this commitment, yet many have problems in implementing it. Four hospital school directors in south metropolitan Chicago found it most difficult to secure qualified faculty. At the invitation of one school, all four decided to join forces in a program which would assist faculty to improve their teaching skills.

One of the schools, the Evangelical School of Nursing, established a fairly effective inservice program for its fifteen faculty members early in 1966. This was found expensive to implement or to expand. A one-day workshop requested by the group cost $225, or $15 per member. When the chairman of continuing education in this school obtained permission to include a neighboring school in order to

Elida L. Mundt is a graduate of Walther Memorial Hospital School of Nursing, Chicago and earned her B.S.N.Ed. and M.Ed. degrees at Loyola University Chicago. Mrs. Mundt is currently administrator of the Evangelical School of Nursing, Oak Lawn, Illinois, the school described as sponsor in this article. This article is reprinted from JONA, January-February, 1971.

reduce costs, it was found that the costs were halved; an even more important result was the enthusiasm of both faculty groups because of the interchange of ideas which the workshop provided. Since there were two other diploma schools nearby with very limited continuing education programs for faculty, the chairman asked permission to invite them also. The administrator of the sponsoring school and hospital again agreed, and also offered the facilities of their school for workshops in order to get a joint program started.

A committee of the four schools met to determine future plans. The name Community Organization of Faculty In-Service (and pronounced "coffee") was adopted and the purpose of the organization agreed upon was "to meet some of the educational needs of the faculty members of four area hospital schools of nursing." The committee consisted of the director and one other faculty member from each school; it later became the Executive Committee on COFI under a federal grant.

A letter of agreement outlined the responsibility of each school for sharing costs, assisting with workshops, and evaluation. Each school polled its faculty to assess interests and needs and the results were pooled to determine topics for eight workshops carried out during the next two years. Evaluation of the joint program after the first year indicated that the workshops had been quite beneficial, but also pointed out greater needs. Schools reported that new faculty members needed "on the job" assistance in developing and teaching nursing courses, in adjusting to the faculty role, in supervising clinical practice, and in evaluating students. These needs, not met through four annual workshops, pointed to the need for a full time program. It was this need which prompted the schools to apply for federal funds for faculty development under the Nurse Training Act of 1964. Our statement of rationale included these assumptions:

1) Effective on-going educational programs are a considerable financial burden for our schools, yet are a necessity to improve our programs.

2) The grass roots problem is not greatly affected by a *general* effort such as periodic workshops on a variety of topics.

3) Instructors need continuing assistance in implementing educational objectives in their courses.

4) New faculty members need more orientation to the teaching role before being assigned full teaching loads.

5) Our schools are able to send very few teachers away for full time study because of staffing numbers. The problem of faculty staffing does not appear to be alleviating and we envision facing like problems during the foreseeable future.

6) It appears necessary for us to work with the faculty members we have, to assist them in improving teaching skills, if we are to continue to offer quality diploma education in nursing.

7) Our schools represent an enrollment of 350-plus students; if we can improve teaching, we will be better preparing these students for professional practice.

8) One full-time project director is needed to implement the program of faculty development we propose. Sharing a director among four schools will reduce inservice costs to each school and sharing of teaching aids and resources should effect additional savings.

9) Working relationship already established among our four schools should enable us to implement effectively the added goals for faculty development we propose. The table of organization accompanying the application defined relationships.

ORGANIZATION OF COFI
NURSE PROJECT GRANT 305

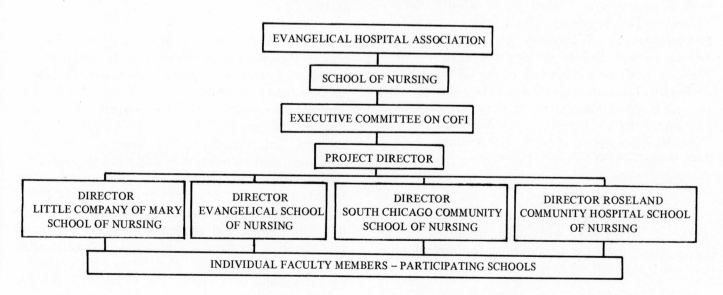

Effective on-going educational programs are a considerable financial burden for our schools, yet essential to program improvement

Funding and Budget

Since our proposal was unique in this area and the few similar programs in other states could furnish little information for us, we found budget estimation difficult. As most administrators know, costs of consultation vary widely and are considerably affected by travel costs and per diem expenses. It is seldom known if local or distant persons must be recruited to fulfill workshop goals. We were somewhat naive about consultation costs. Joint programs prior to the grant had ranged from $75.00 to $200.00 per day (less than $5.00 per member). When an early one day workshop under the grant resulted in a bill of $400.00 from a local consultant we were stunned. We had obtained only an oral agreement, and had not even conceived of including planning time and post-evaluation procedures of the consultant in our budget. Since that time, all commitments have been obtained in writing and workshop goals have been specifically detailed. Despite the problems which estimating costs posed for us in advance, we closely approximated our budget a year and a half later. It was necessary during both the first and second years to secure approval for transfer of funds from one budget category to another to attain our objectives.

Pamphlets that were helpful in obtaining a federal project grant were *Public Health Service Grants for Training Projects,* and *Instructions for the Preparation and Submission of Applications for Special Project Grants for Improvement in Nurse Training.* Both are publications of the US Department of Health, Education and Welfare. Our schools aked for and received consultation from the Project Grants Section of HEW and gained information needed to complete the application for federal funding.

Organization

Rules and regulations for the Executive Committee on COFI were written and approved by that body. These provided a framework for implementing the grant and outlined five functions:

1) to approve job descriptions of the project director and secretary

2) to approve guidelines for use of the project director in implementing the grant

3) to act upon recommendations submitted by individual schools through their representatives

4) to recommend purchases and expenditures in accord with grant provisions

5) to evaluate the progress of the grant bi-monthly and at the completion of the project period.

The grant provided funds for setting up an office at the Evangelical School of Nursing. Any program requires certain office and bookkeeping procedures, whether kept by the hospital or the project staff. In order to plan future programs, travel, etc., it is necessary to have a running knowledge of what has been spent and what remains in each budget category. This pointed up the necessity of finding a secretary with some bookkeeping skills. Records kept in the COFI office included the school catalog and curriculum of each school, a record of the background and experience of each member, a collection of books on curriculum and instruction, journals and reports of workshop and institutes (written or taped) for loan to members. Teaching aids required to implement workshops and programs were purchased and also housed in the COFI office.

Staff

Job descriptions were formulated for the project director and secretary and approved by the Executive Committee. Qualifications for the project director were described as follows: a registered professional nurse with an appropriate masters degree, a minimum of five years experience in both teaching and administrative aspects of nursing education, and an interest in and skills necessary for implementing the program of inservice education described in the project grant application. She would be responsible to the Executive Committee on COFI and would plan and implement workshops, orient new members to their faculty roles, and assist other members with instructional problems when requested by individuals or schools. The Committee decided that one COFI member met these qualifications and that her familiarity with all four schools would enable her to work well with the faculty members. The director chosen had been on the staff of the sponsoring school, chairman of their continuing education committee, and chairman of COFI since its inception; she had initiated the idea of joint service. Her previous position had included consultation for nursing schools throughout the state as Assistant Coordinator of Nursing Education in Illinois.

Funds provided under the grant enabled the director to seek consultation as necessary to implement the program, not only for major workshops but also for monthly two-hour educational programs. Consultants were obtained from headquarters staff of the National League for Nursing as well as from colleges and universities throughout the US. Local educators, nurses and non-nurses were utilized to implement the goals of monthly programs. Qualification of all workshop consultants required prior approval by the Project Grants Section of HEW.

Public Relations and Publicity

A requirement of HEW to grantees (schools) is that project grants be publicized and that results which would be of assistance to others be made available. Many schools of nursing in 1968–1969 were searching for answers to problems of faculty inservice, and we did share our first years' activities and evaluation with them, both individually and to a large audience at a professional meeting. We believe that our efforts in publicizing the grant are directly responsible for similar programs now being discussed, one in another area of the city and a second in another area of Illinois. Further, by making the community aware of our efforts to improve our schools of nursing, we were encouraging their continued support of diploma education and promoting recruitment.

We hoped our efforts to include other hospital personnel in our programs (such as head nurses and supervisors) would encourage them to improve their own inservice programs and point out the benefits of joint planning. We found that workshop consultants publicized our program too; one referred a faculty group at some distance to find out about our project. A newsletter was published to inform members of coming programs; it shared information about curricula and programs of each school and helped to promote a feeling of fellowship among members.

Establishing Objectives

The Executive Committee formulated objectives for the program. It was decided that these would necessarily be broad since the needs of our schools and individual members varied considerably. Of our 55–60 members, some 25 percent were beginning instructors and another 25 percent had several years of teaching experience. The remaining 50 percent were members with five or more years of teaching experience. This latter group included seven with masters degrees. Most of these members had graduated eight or more years ago; despite considerable experience, many were not up-to-date on modern teaching and measurement methods, curriculum development, etc. It became quite evident that both new and experienced members needed information on current curriculum concepts and teaching methods, which led us to adopt as an objective: to keep faculty abreast of new trends in nursing and nursing education. We had already experienced the benefits of sharing ideas and felt this should be a continuing goal which was stated in a second objective: to facilitate the exchange of ideas and teaching methods. With a full-time project director this could be enhanced as ideas useful in one school were brought to other schools she worked with. Believing that one outcome of the project should be to help our members become the leaders in nursing we so desperately need (the top priority revealed by the Illinois Study Commission on Nursing), we formulated a third objective: to provide a means for personal and professional growth.

Implementing the Objectives

Working to meet our goals took a little different form in each agency. When a number of new faculty members joined the staff in a school, weekly discussion programs were held on the whole gamut of nursing education topics, such as: (1) the role of the faculty member in the diploma program; (2) the

One objective was to keep faculty abreast of new trends in nursing and nursing education

status of nursing education in Illinois; (3) implementing the educational philosophy; (4) formulating course objectives; (5) implementing objectives in theory and clinical practice; (6) course outlines and lesson plans; (7) teaching methods; (8) evaluation; (9) National League for Nursing criteria; (10) research in nursing; (11) the responsibility of the professional person to the community.

Suggested readings accompanied these programs and all new faculty were provided with a bibliography of publications helpful to them. COFI library books were loaned to new as well as to regular members. New members were expected to attend weekly inservice programs and a number of experienced members elected to attend also. Classes were open to all teachers and topics were publicized in advance so that persons desiring refresher information could receive it. Sometimes sessions included taped segments of workshop content from outside programs; we also discussed content from our own workshops which needed clarification. In one school there had been no new faculty for several years; their members chose to have the weekly programs to bring them up to date on new ideas and curriculum methods and, as a result, decided they needed to revise their school's philosophy and objectives; this task became the focus of that school's programs for several months.

When evaluation at year-end showed weekly programs to have been too time consuming for our schools, we changed to monthly joint programs on topics related to an annual theme, and engaged a consultant for many of these. The Vimcet filmstrip-tape series on teaching was used in the second year for orientation of new members and in some of the educational programs for all faculty. Orientation of new members was scheduled during the summer and/or scheduled individually in free periods in early fall.

Our overall theme for a three-year period was "The Role of the Faculty Member in Implementing the School Program." Each of three subtopics, curriculum development and teaching methods, counseling and guidance, and evaluation, became the focus for a year. The needs of our members were made known to each consultant and planning sessions

were held in advance of workshops. The project director, the Executive Committee, and the consultant were all involved in designing programs appropriate for our group.

For example, prior to a workshop on implementing the professional philosophy and objectives, we assessed the number and timeliness of courses our members had had on this subject and decided that most could verbalize Bloom's *Taxonomy* but needed help in writing specific behavioral objectives. We also introduced the subject of Affective Objectives since these are less familiar and would challenge our better prepared members.

Our assessments of member needs were not always accurate but they did improve as the project developed. We now find that our members grasp new information readily and schedule time carefully to avoid covering familiar content. The entire second year focused on Guidance and Counseling. We began with the newly-admitted student and, with the help of consultants, explored what the 1969 student was like and how the faculty member could help in his (her) adjustment. We discussed ways to increase enrollment by recruiting disadvantaged students and licensed practical nurses; consultants reported on their experiences in working with these groups. A two-day counseling workshop was planned with a consultant for every ten members. Each member role-played counselor or counselee in exploring common student problems from our own schools, under the direction of expert counselors.

A topic for the current year is Evaluation: for two workshop days we are focusing on Test Construction and Clinical Evaluation. Although this is an "old hat" topic for most teachers, it was chosen by our members because several of the schools are involved in efforts to introduce pass-fail criteria in their courses and it should afford new information for their task.

Frequently the details of a program were only tentatively scheduled in advance so that programs could change to meet the needs of members. On occasion group leaders met with workshop consultants the evening before a program in order to insure that a productive day would follow.

Nearly every workshop involved small group activity and we rotated group leadership roles among members. Orientation to all workshops began with an annual schedule which was added to when workshop goals were further discussed in the project newsletter and completed when individual programs were sent out several weeks in advance. Included with the program was a suggested bibliography to be used in preparation for participation, and a curriculum vita of our consultant(s). Attendance at workshops has been required of faculty; workshop days are free of student's classes and COFI workshop days are also free days for students.

There are now four major workshops a year and a monthly joint two-hour program for *all* faculty. The orientation for new members continues as described. The project director is available to faculty in each school each week to assist faculty as they may request. A sample weeks' schedule might include: (1) showing a filmstrip-tape on writing objectives to a new faculty member; (2) assisting a teacher to write her first objective examination; (3) evaluating a revised course outline; (4) discussing part-time courses available with an interested member; (5) attending a curriculum committee meeting when objectives are being revised; (6) assisting an instructor to evaluate students; or (7) counseling a member about future education.

Talking with members about continuing education opportunities was considered one of our most important activities. A monthly program on graduate education further stimulated our members to continue their education. As a means of meeting one of our objectives, reports of workshops, institutes, meetings, etc., were taped, summarized by the project director and circulated to all members in order that all would be informed of new ideas and trends. On several occasions a member of the Executive Committee also attended a workshop or meeting, under the sponsorship of the grant. Each school was asked to report the on-going educational needs of its faculty at meetings of the Executive Committee so that schedules could be coordinated among schools.

There are problems of scheduling when four schools are involved. We did manage to clear days for major workshops and monthly programs and coor-

dinated requests of individual schools at committee meetings. The time of inservice programs is still reportedly inconvenient for some and we have been unable to solve this problem.

Among our growing pains were problems of arrangements. Members prefer to learn close to home, we found, and were sometimes critical of workshops held at some distance because of the travel involved. Grant funds, also, do not cover food costs; administrators planning joint workshops will find luncheons in metropolitan areas will add about $3.00 per person to the cost of programs. Members were sometimes dissatisfied with luncheons and arrangments, despite a variety of settings chosen for workshops.

Our schools are from two to ten miles apart; though this represented considerable weekly travel for the project director, it was possible to reach the farthest school within an hour. We have been able to share teaching aids among our schools too. The audio-visual department of one school (Little Company of Mary) was used to prepare a video-tape for a workshop program; we found it possible to share other equipment, on occasion, which resulted in the saving of rental fees.

Evaluation

Assessment of our efforts was a continuous activity. In the early days of the project it gave direction to future planning for both budget and program. It provided evidence, at the end of each year, that we were meeting our objectives and induced HEW to renew our application for a second and a third year.

At first we evaluated each workshop in terms of overall COFI objectives; we later revised this when results of evaluations became unwieldy to summarize. Also, activities other than workshops assisted in meeting these goals and it was felt, after the first year, that it was not necessary to restate the objectives as frequently.

Workshop evaluation results were sent to all members and were discussed at Executive Committee meetings. We further shared results with our consultants, following workshops.

At the end of each year an opinionnaire was

The larger the group, the less the per-person cost of individual educational programs

completed by each member. A summary of opinions was utilized in planning programs for the next year. Each member received a copy of the summary so that he would be familiar with the overall reaction to our program.

The project director was continually asking the Executive Committee and individual members to suggest ways in which the program could be of greater service and asked opinions of members in informal contacts. Many of the most profitable suggestions came from those who questioned its progress. When several members voiced the opinion that COFI ought to be more of an instrument for change in our schools, both project director and Executive Committee became a little anxious. We decided together that as a voluntary agency we could not implement change but were perhaps responsible for *influencing* more desirable changes. Realizing that changes come about through people, we tried to involve people who could make changes. We began to hear frequent discussions about personnel policies during the second year, particularly about variations in faculty work load which existed among our schools. A request from members to have an open meeting about personnel policies was declined by the Executive Committee; however, it was agreed to investigate at the Committee level. The project director surveyed other schools and gathered data on faculty policies which was shared at a committee meeting. When efforts were made by each school to meet competitive policies, group concern was lessened. Following a program on Student Organizations in which faculty members had an opportunity to discuss concepts of freedom and responsibility in education, significant changes in school policy were made in several of our schools. Perhaps COFI has been an instrument for change after all.

Summary

That COFI has met a need, we are convinced. It has been responsible for encouraging continuing education. Seven of eighteen faculty members in one school alone were enrolled in courses during the past two years, nine out of sixteen this year. Four COFI members left for full time graduate study and four more are planning to enter graduate programs full time within the next year or two. About a third of our members have been counseled about available courses and we have supplied references for some who made application.

One school closed at the end of the second year because of financial and recruitment problems. The librarian of this school expressed in a letter her comments about what COFI had meant to their school and how it would continue to influence each member in her future work.

Former members now in graduate school report they feel better prepared than their peers as a result of COFI programs and are able to use reports and information gained in current course projects. A few of our members have stated the content of COFI programs approximates what they are getting in graduate courses and asked why credit cannot be offered for COFI programs.

Pattern for Others

Recently a faculty member who was leaving told me that she would miss COFI very much and thought that she would work to get one started in a school to which she was moving, some distance away. We hope she will and we know others who might do the same thing someday.

Some have had the impression that our project is joint inservice for *staff nurses* of four hospitals. Though probably easier to administer for a faculty group we would say, "Why not?" The concept of sharing is the important ingredient. Most hospitals have inservice programs, but within their own walls. It is much more stimulating to meet with groups from other agencies, and to discover that we have *common* problems. The interchange of ideas is one of the enjoyable aspects of joint inservice.

Cost is another factor. Consultants are more readily available to larger groups. Often a well-qualified person is extremely busy and may well decline an invitation to address a small group, but might accept if the needs of many could be served at a workshop. The larger the group, the less the per-person cost of individual educational programs, an important consideration in an era when inservice is an absolute must for all health workers.

It would appear beneficial for nearby hospitals to share information on policies, procedures, record forms, orientation, philosophy and objectives, and even (if they dare) personnel policies. Perhaps turnover, common to all hospitals, could be reduced when salary and fringe benefits are more closely approximated among hospitals in the same areas as a result of joint discussions.

It may be that staff numbers are too large to accommodate several agencies at one program. It would still be possible for supervisors, inservice directors, head nurses, or administrators to have joint programs. Perhaps an agency could plan one program monthly for various levels or specialty areas and invite representatives of other health agencies to join them. If this were started, I believe joint inservice would sell itself. Many nurses do not attend meetings of their professional organizations because of distance, not knowing others, etc. Perhaps they would be willing to discuss topics of interest closer to home, in their own or in a neighboring hospital.

Our experience in COFI has led us to believe that joint inservice works. It is less *costly* (our own costs per workshop were reduced from $15.00 per person to less than $5.00). It can offer better programs because outstanding leaders can be secured for a larger group and, as our members report repeatedly, it is more challenging and interesting to meet with people whose ideas you haven't already heard every day at work.

Two schools of nursing not members of COFI are sending a few faculty members to our programs during this year. They hope to get a similar program started in their area. We have letters from others who state a similar goal. Why not? we ask.

The most rewarding part of inservice and of our project has been to witness the growth of individual members. Some of our members would not even ask a question of the speaker at early workshops and contributed nothing to small group discussions. Now they are group leaders and assume leadership roles in their own schools. I recall a workshop in which the consultant preferred we not select group leaders in advance; members would gravitate to groups of their choice and a "natural" leader would emerge, he felt. We waited for some fifteen minutes of an hour and a half session and no one emerged. Finally he pointed out a potential leader to me and I, not willing to wait longer, asked this person if she would *please* serve as leader. Today she and most of our other members volunteer readily and do a good job as group leaders.

There is much potential ability in any nursing staff, whether it is a faculty or nursing service group. Our job as inservice educators is to bring this out, to facilitate the learning and growth of our members so that they can assume leadership in the profession. We, as teachers, have an awesome task. As Henry Brooks Adams, noted educator, has stated, "A teacher affects eternity; he can never tell where his influence stops."

If you embark on a venture like ours, you may find you have a lion by the tail. You know what happens when you light a candle—fire spreads.

REFERENCES

1. GALLAGHER, ANNA HELEN. *Educational Administration in Nursing.* New York, The Macmillan Co., 1965.

The grant ended in 1971 but continues under the private support of three hospital schools, two of whom were included in the project grant from its inception. The sponsoring school under the grant continues as the legal sponsor. A series of workshops are jointly sponsored annually and schools continue to cooperate in various ways to support diploma education in nursing. This is further described in another article based on an oral presentation at the 1974 annual meeting of the Council of Diploma Programs entitled "Continuing Education and Self Learning for Faculties As Seen by a Nursing School Administrator". The article appears in the just released NLN publication *The Changing Role.*

The Clinical Specialist: Her Role in Staff Development

By Margaret Smith Byrne

Inherent growth needs of nursing staff must be met to insure staff growth and achievement of quality patient care. Certain leadership skills insure the meeting of inherent growth needs. A nursing clinical specialist who understands and practices these skills with staff can provide the stimulus to achieve increased quality of patient care, more efficient use of time and materials, higher staff productivity, and a higher turnover of patients.

Health professionals as well as consumers are becoming more verbal about the inadequacies of the health care system and it is clear that improvement is necessary. There are many roads to improvement of the system, one of which is the proper use of the clinical specialist. With her role properly developed the clinical specialist can effect many changes both in and out of the hospital setting.

As a clinical specialist for the past year and a half in a medical-surgical setting, my objective has been to improve interaction between the staff and the patient. This implies that the staff must do some things differently than before I came into the setting. The goals have been: more involvement of the patient in his own care, more evidence of planning for his

care, more concern about what will happen when he leaves the hospital, and more cooperation among health team members.

Evidence of increased involvement of the patient in his own care is demonstrated when the staff have a patient-care planning conference and invite the patient and his family to attend; they can then develop a care plan in which the patient has participated. When staff members make walking rounds at the change of shift and include the patient in their discussion of current medical plans, changes observed in his condition and needs identified by patient or staff, they are involving the patient in his own care.

Evidence of current care planning is demonstrated by nursing history interviews, done by the staff when the patient is admitted. During this interview, information is collected from the patient so that a care plan can be developed. During the interview the staff member also orients the patient to the unit and encourages his cooperation in planning with the staff. Further evidence of planning is seen on new and updated care plans for each patient and daily patient planning conferences.

Evidence of concern about post-hospital care is demonstrated by increased awareness of the staff regarding such things as the patient's knowledge of his disease, the patient's environmental surroundings, the patient's social-economic conditions and the family members' response to the illness.

Margaret Smith Byrne received a B.S.N. from the University of Iowa and an M.S. degree in community health nursing from the University of California. She has done post master's work with a second clinical area in psychiatric nursing at the University of California and has completed work on an M.S. in organizational psychology at California State University, San Francisco. Ms. Byrne was a clinical specialist at the Veterans Administration Hospital in San Francisco when this article was written. This article is reprinted from JONA, January-February, 1971.

Health team cooperation is evidenced by appropriate referrals from the nursing staff to the social worker, dietician, and psychologist soon after admission of the patient. This practice has facilitated discharge planning by early involvement of allied team members. The nursing staff look forward to weekly multidisciplinary conferences because they have more to contribute than in the past, and because they increase their knowledge of their patients by sharing information with the total health team. Because the nursing staff have increased knowledge and awareness of the patient, the physicians in this kind of setting state that they have more time to focus on the medical problems of the patient; this is further evidence of greater health team cooperation.

The clinical specialist, to be truly effective, must function through others and can be more effective if certain basic notions are recognized. To begin with, many factors have been identified over the years which contribute to the productivity and satisfaction of employees in any organization. These factors apply to nursing or to any other part of the health system, just as they apply to industrial systems. Employee needs are one set of factors, leadership skills another.

Employee Needs

In any group of employees, it is possible to identify two sets of needs: deficiency reduction needs and inherent growth needs.[1] Herzberg states that these needs have independent and distinct characteristics and that to be met each requires different organizational behavior.[2]

Deficiency needs may be met by behavior which improves working conditions, improves salary, changes policy, and the like.

Inherent growth needs may be met by behavior which acknowledges achievement, gives recognition and responsibility, provides for advancement, expands knowledge, etc. It is my view that meeting the inherent growth needs of staff at all levels is the major function of the clinical specialist. She must provide growth stimulation for all members of the unit including the supervisory and administrative staff.

Leadership Skills

Bowers and Seashore identify four leadership skills which stimulate growth.[3] These skills are: support, interaction facilitation, goal emphasis, and work facilitation.

Support is behavior which increases or maintains the individual's sense of personal worth and importance in the context of group activity. For example, I meet in various groups, listen to the ideas offered by any group member and acknowledge them as valuable. Recently I have worked with a planning group composed of registered nurses and nursing assistants. The nursing assistants expressed the desire to assume more responsibility for patient care. Rather then dismiss this idea as some members of the group were inclined to do, I encouraged the entire group to listen to the feelings expressed about wanting more responsibility and to the ideas presented for increasing the nursing assistants' responsibilities.

Interaction facilitation is behavior which creates or maintains a network of interpersonal relationships among group members. The objective is to create an atmosphere in which direct expression of response one to the other is acceptable. If a given response is unfavorable, I help the individuals discuss what they are feeling and thinking and attempt to move them toward a better understanding of each other's subjective feelings and objective responses. For example, I may ask someone in a group for clarification of an idea or feeling he has expressed, or I may respond to the emotional level of the whole group and explore with them their responses to the situation.

Goal emphasis is behavior which creates, changes, or gains member acceptance of group goals. The group I worked with developed goals and objectives for their unit. They used the goals for the entire nursing service. Their guidelines were their own knowledge and feelings about the kind of care a patient should receive. As they then developed roles, an idea, presented by a nursing assistant, to develop a co-team leader role, was accepted. The idea was that the nursing assistant assume joint responsibility with the professional nurse to make daily patient assignments; identify problems in patient care, especially

Effective leadership leads to group cohesiveness, common goals, shared responsibility, and a sense of individual achievement

physical; identify staff problems or dissatisfactions and conduct team conferences focused on identified problems. The registered nurse was to assume a guidance and teaching role as she worked with the co-team leader. The group needed much help discussing this particular role, designing it to fit their objectives, developing the responsibility for the nursing assistant and the ultimate accountability of the registered nurse. I helped them work through the development of their goals, objectives, and roles.

Work facilitation is behavior which provides effective work methods and facilitates the accomplishment of group goals. During the planning phase of the above-mentioned group, I contributed knowledge about group process which other group members did not have. This knowledge facilitated the accomplishment of the task, which was to plan their approach to patient care. Had I not been available to them, they would have been less productive and spent more time disagreeing and coping with their feelings. The planning phase is now completed; I work with groups of staff members to develop their skills with interviewing, patient care planning, and effective work organization.

For the development of staff to occur a proper climate must be established. This growth climate follows from proper exercise of management skills and behaviors such as have been discussed. With leadership, each staff member will grow and develop according to his or her own needs. If the goals of nursing service are clear and understandable for the group, this process of individual growth will occur in conjunction with organizational goals.

Effective leadership will lead to group cohesiveness, the establishment of common goals, the sharing of responsibility, mutual cooperation and recognition, plus a sense of individual achievement because everyone contributes in his own right.

This process of learning and growth must occur at the unit, supervisory, and administrative levels. It is an erroneous assumption of many nursing services that only unit level staff need development.

Likert[4] would probably call this approach to staff development participative group management. Dr. Likert states that in any management system there are certain variables which can be differentiated

into three categories: causal, intervening, and end result. Manipulation of causal variables causes differences in intervening and end result variables. Likert diagrams various approaches to management showing the results of different causal variables. Figure one illustrates this approach as applied to a nursing unit.

FIGURE 1

If a Nursing Service has:

Well organized plan of operation
High performance goals
High technical competence
(manager or staff assistants)

and if the supervisor manages via:

	Authoritarian Systems e.g., uses	Group Participative Systems e.g., uses
Causal Variables	direct hierarchial pressure for results, punishment, competition	supportive relationships, group methods of supervision recognition, reward, responsibility

her nursing unit will display:

Intervening Variables	less group loyalty	greater group loyalty
	lower performance goals	higher performance goals
	greater conflict and less cooperation	greater cooperation
	less technical assistance to peers	more technical assistance to peers
	greater feeling of unreasonable pressure	less feeling of unreasonable pressure
	less favorable attitudes toward supervisor	more favorable attitudes toward supervisor
	lower motivation to produce	higher motivation to produce

and her nursing unit will display:

End-result Variables	low turnover of patients	high turnover of patients
	low quality of patient care	high quality of patient care
	high waste of time and materials	less waste of time and materials
	low productivity of staff	high productivity of staff

In an authoritarian system of management, Dr. Likert suggests the causal variables may be: decisions made at the top level, use of punishment rather than reward, sparing recognition, and a single-minded management orientation toward production. The intervening variables would be low group loyalty, low performance goals, unfavorable attitudes toward management, and low motivation to produce.

In a group participative system of management one would expect, as causal variables, encouragement of decisions at the working level, rewards for achievement, recognition and responsibility for subordinates, and high value placed on group action and group feelings. The intervening variables would be high group loyalty, high performance goals, favorable attitudes toward management, and high motivation to produce.

Where the end result variables in an authoritarian system of management are high costs, lower quality and volume; in group participative management it is assumed the end result variables are increased quality of patient care, more efficient use of time and materials, higher staff productivity, and higher turnover of patients. This assumption, based on Likert's theory of management, is currently being studied by the author.

The role of the clinical specialist is to stimulate a group participative approach, using the leadership skills stressed earlier: support, interaction facilitation, goal emphasis, and work facilitation.

This approach must be initiated at the causal variable level. Intervention at any other variable will not produce lasting change in the system. This approach meets the inherent growth needs of the staff and stimulates their productivity and creativity in meeting the needs of patients.

The clinical specialist with a specific case load is focussing on the work facilitation aspect of leadership and the other three elements are bound to suffer. All the leadership elements must receive their due. Otherwise, while patient care by the specialist may be excellent, the staff will function no differently in relation to the other patients.

Assignment of specific case loads to clinical specialists is a narrow approach to hospital management and to the welfare of patients. Clinical specialists must be utilized in a way that promotes the growth of *all* staff members to the benefit of *all* patients.

REFERENCES

1. MASLOW, A. "Deficiency Motivation and Growth Motivation," ed. by M. R. Jones, *Nebraska Symposium on Motivation*. Lincoln, University of Nebraska Press, 1955.
2. HERZBÈRG, F. *Work and the Nature of Man*. Cleveland, World Publishing Co., 1966.
3. BOWERS, D. and SEASHORE, S. "Predicting Organizational Effectiveness with a Four-Factor Theory of Leadership," *Administrative Science Quarterly* 11:2, Sept. 1966.
4. LIKERT, R. *The Human Organization: Its Management and Value*. New York, McGraw-Hill Book Co., 1967.

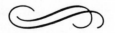

Bridging the Gap Between

by Myrna L. Armstrong

An orientation unit was created to provide guided learning experiences and to ease into the work environment new graduates with varied skills and educational preparation for nursing.

At the time this article was written, **Myrna Armstrong,** B.S.N., M.S., was surgical inservice coordinator, Thomas Jefferson University Hospital, Philadelphia, Pennsylvania. She is currently residing in California. This article is reprinted from JONA, November-December, 1974.

Nursing service administrators are becoming increasingly aware of the problems and frustrations generated in the patient care setting by and for new graduates coming to the work environment from a wide variety of nursing schools and three levels in nursing education. New graduates from associate degree, diploma, and baccalaureate nursing programs beginning their first jobs after graduation have been exposed to different kinds and amounts of experience in a hospital setting. Representatives of these three levels cannot be considered equal either in their educational preparation for practice or in their ability to function effectively in the service setting.

Many new graduates begin work with a wealth of knowledge but limited clinical experience; they are more educationally oriented than service oriented to the role and responsibilities they are expected to assume. Since the employing hospital or institution expects and usually needs these new nurses to fill staff vacancies as soon as possible, the first experience as full-time members of the nursing staff can become a traumatic and frustrating experience both for the newcomers and for those with whom they work. Frustration, which in turn produces disillusionment for those new graduates who find that they are unable to cope with their responsibilities, frequently results in termination of employment as well. A by-product of this situation, of course, is a never-ending high turnover of nursing personnel that has caused nursing service administrators to become increasingly concerned about the need to bridge the gap between graduation and employment and to find an effective method to ease new graduates with varied educational backgrounds into the nursing service for which they have been prepared.

Where does the nurse administrator begin? Traditionally the employing institution provides an orientation period for new personnel to prepare them for the practical and technical aspects of the various duties and responsibilities assigned to them. The orientation period, however, is usually brief and too geared to the policies and procedures peculiar to the employing institution to provide the time and opportunity for new graduates to practice techniques or to develop the skill and ability necessary to function effectively on a service unit. Although the inservice or staff development department has an active role to play in preparing new graduates for their assignments during the orientation

Graduation and Employment

period, an individualized yet flexible orientation program is also required to meet both the staffing needs of the employer and the ongoing practice needs of new graduates beginning work with limited clinical experience.

How does a small group of staff development personnel coordinate new graduate activities on many different service units and still provide meaningful experiences for new nurses beginning practice with different educational backgrounds as well as with different kinds and amounts of clinical experience? A review of the literature suggests such ideas as an orientation unit, rotation of new graduates to all clinical areas, and internship. After considering all these ideas, we chose the orientation unit to deal with the problem at Thomas Jefferson University Hospital.

Planning the Orientation Unit

In 1972, Thomas Jefferson University Hospital created a decentralized nursing service with assistant directors responsible for the administrative duties of particular clinical areas. Figure 1 shows the organization of the nursing department. This type of organization structure has created a more autonomous feeling within each clinical area. Within this organization, our staff development department consists of two divisions, both of which play an active role in the development of graduate personnel. Responsible to the assistant director of research and development is the central

staff development group. This division is responsible for presenting to all nursing employees the hospital's nursing philosophy and personnel policies, and for introducing these employees to the problem-oriented record and to an overview of the various support services within the hospital. The other division is the decentralized group, composed of medical and surgical inservice coordinators who assist their respective assistant directors and supervisors in planning nursing personnel development through education. These inservice coordinators have four main functions within their clinical areas. First, with the use of an inservice committee chosen from all levels of nursing personnel within the department, the inservice coordinator selects and conducts formal monthly education programs for the registered nurse, practical nurse, and nursing assistant. Second, the inservice coordinator evaluates patient care needs, generates and participates in team conferences, and assists head nurses in the implementation of new programs through education. Third, the inservice coordinator is responsible for the orientation of all newly employed registered and practical nurses to the patient unit. Fourth, the inservice coordinator works closely with instructors from the three Thomas Jefferson University schools of nursing (baccalaureate, diploma, and practical), as well as with other professional departments and schools, in providing the staff with educational opportunities having the ultimate goal of better

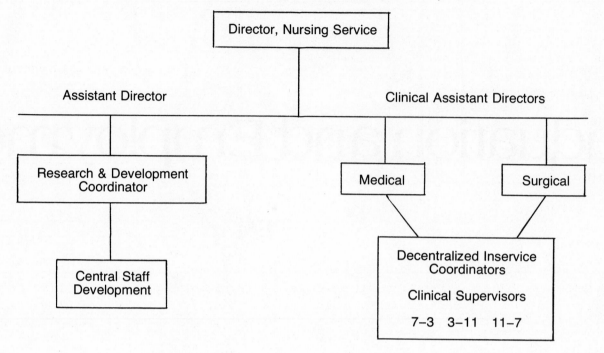

FIGURE 1. Organization chart for staff development department

Director, Nursing Service

Assistant Director

Clinical Assistant Directors

Research & Development Coordinator

Medical

Surgical

Central Staff Development

Decentralized Inservice Coordinators

Clinical Supervisors

7–3   3–11   11–7

patient care and development of personnel at all levels.

Our objective, then, was to create an individually guided orientation program for our newly graduated employees and at the same time to introduce them to specific hospital policies and procedures. By using the concept of an orientation unit, we believed that inservice coordinators could assess the nursing skills the new graduates brought with them, provide better and controlled experiences, allow new personnel to grow in nursing skills, and develop leadership qualities. The duration of the orientation period would be a minimum of four weeks, after which the new graduates would be moved to their assigned medical or surgical units. We felt at this time that newly employed graduates from our own nursing education programs could be assigned directly to their permanent units since they were familiar with the hospital, and that only new graduates from schools other than Thomas Jefferson University Hospital schools of nursing should be assigned to the proposed orientation units. The rationale for this decision was to be evaluated later by the head nurses and the inservice coordinators.

Selection of the Unit

Because the first few weeks of employment can create a lasting impression for the new nurse, the determination of which patient units should be utilized as orientation units was an important consideration. Each unit's head nurse, her graduate staff, and the type of clinical service provided, all had to be evaluated. The administrative atmosphere of a proposed patient unit had to be one of a flexible and creative, but organized, nature. The head nurse had to be a willing instructor, and other staff members had to be deemed good role models in order to present to the new graduates an image of a workable and responsible nursing service. The patient unit also had to provide the kind of clinical experience necessary to care for the types of patients the new graduates would be working with in their permanent units; otherwise these newcomers might become restless at the idea that they would have to learn to care for another type of patient later.

In selecting the patient units for our project, the inservice coordinators and assistant directors discussed the concept of the orientation project with the nursing staff permanently assigned to the areas being considered. This discussion included the goals of the project, the staff's function as role models, and the teaching responsibilities of each level of personnel on the unit. Staff members on the units were asked if they wanted to take part in this project. Both the medical and the surgical units selected were eager to participate, for they felt that the program would be a learning experience for them, stimulating their present nursing conferences, care plans, and patient care. The nursing staff did ask if the increase in personnel because of the newly employed graduate nurses on an orientation unit would result in their being asked more frequently to work on other patient care units. It was decided by the assistant director that the staffing pattern would remain the same on both medical and

surgical units to facilitate the goals of the orientation units and to provide the new graduates with a readily available resource group.

Orientation Unit Activities

After finding an appropriate environment, the inservice coordinators began to formulate a tentative plan of guided experiences for the new graduate nurses that would apply the theory obtained in the nursing educational program to the working environment. These experiences would include patient care, the administration of medications, and team leadership; the time spent on these activities would depend on the individual new graduate. A schedule outlining the various month-long orientation activities was prepared for each newly employed graduate nurse and was posted at the orientation unit to provide both the new nurse and the head nurse with knowledge of the day's activities (see Figure 2).

The new nurse's first week on the orientation unit was spent delivering patient care, developing care plans, and becoming accustomed to the problem-oriented medical record. The inservice coordinators were present on the patient unit during this time to make assignments, to assist in the new graduates' adjustment to the work environment, and to act as a resource person. By working closely with these

FIGURE 2. Thomas Jefferson University Hospital Nursing Service staff development—orientation schedule

Name _____   Date _____

The following schedule has been created to assist you in becoming familiar with the Clinical Area in the hospital. The Inservice Coordinator will be adjusting your orientation according to your nursing education and experience. Please feel free to contact her at any time.

		Monday	Tuesday	Wednesday	Thursday	Friday
1	OFF	Date 8–1 P.M. Central Orientation; 1–4:30 P.M. Introduction to Orientation Unit	Date 7–10:30 A.M. Team Member 1 Patient; 10:30–12 Central Orientation Problem-Oriented Chart; 12:30–3:30 **Team Member** Admission, if possible	Date 7–3:30 3 Patients Admission of Patient Discharge Procedure	Date 7–3:30 4 Patients Team Conference Care Plans	Date 7–3:30 4 Patients Care Plans; 2 P.M. Conference with Inservice Coordinator
2	OFF	7–3:30 4 Patients Doctors' Rounds Team Conference	Team Member 7–12:30 4 Pts. Team Conference 1–3:30; Central Orientation 1–1:30 Philosophy with Assist. Director; 1:30–2:30 Cardiopulmon. Resusc.; 2:30–3:30 Max Cart	Team Member 7–11:30 4 Pts. Team Conference Doctor's Rounds; Central Orientation 12–1 Incident Reports; 1–2 Fire Safety; 2–3:30 Tour—Hospital	Team Member 7–11:30 ½ day c̄ Pt. Unit Clerk; Central Orientation 12–1 Aux-Clerical Duties; 1–2 A-V Shunt; 2–3:30 IV Therapy	Team Member 7–2 P.M. Review Med. System 2 P.M. Conference with Inservice Coordinator
3	OFF	Medications for 2 teams	Team Member 7–1 Meds for floor; Central Orientation 1:30–2:30 Inhalation Rx; 2:30–3:30 Respiratory Care	Team Member 7–1 2 Patients Transcription orders; Central Orientation 1:30–2:30 Monitor & Care; 2:30–3:30 Peri Dialysis	Team Member 7–12 3 Patients Transcription orders; 12:30–1:30 Isolation Policies; 1:30–2;30 Pharmacy; 2:30–3:30 X-ray	Team Member 7–12:30 Observe Team Leader 1–2 Cardiac Cath. 2 P.M. Conference c̄ Inservice Coordinator
4	OFF	7–3:30 Team Leader without Medications (function with another leader, if possible)	7–3:30 Team Leader with Meds.	7–3:30 Team Leader with Meds.	7–3:30 With Head Nurse to observe duties	7–3:30 Team Member 2 P.M. Conference with Inservice Coordinator
5				To permanently assigned unit		

45

graduates, the coordinator found it possible to evaluate them and to adjust floor assignments individually before too many frustrating crises occurred.

During the afternoons of the second and third weeks, the new graduates attended introductory classes to the various departments of the hospital. We felt that new graduates were better able to understand the introductory classes conducted or coordinated by the central orientation division after having been exposed to the working environment. Also, during the second and third weeks of the orientation period, the inservice coordinators planned for the new graduate's participation in team conferences, in more patient care, in doctors' rounds, and in guided experiences in administering medications.

Each new graduate also spent half a day with the patient unit clerks during the second week, developing a view toward an understanding of the many clerical duties performed on the unit. Time spent delivering patient care, administering medications, attending orientation classes, transcribing doctors' orders, and working with the various auxiliary nursing personnel was designed to give the new graduates a foundation for better coordination of the tasks they would be expected to organize when they became team leaders.

During the fourth and final week on the unit the new graduates functioned as team leaders, coordinating the activities they had experienced during the previous weeks. Depending on the individual, this plan was modified according to practice needs and educational background.

The Evaluation Process

Evaluation conferences were held weekly with each new graduate. During these conferences it was stressed that the inservice coordinator could anticipate many of the new graduates' orientation and practice needs, but communication on their part was also essential to their growth.

A three-section questionnaire, designed to evelute the new graduates' performance in various stages of orientation to the hospital, was prepared. The first section was a skills inventory covering the various nursing equipment and procedures each newcomer had or had not worked with. This section was completed by the new nurses upon their arrival on the orientation unit, and supervision and practical application of nursing experience were provided when necessary.

All new graduates were asked to complete the second part of the questionnaire after four weeks on the orientation unit and before going to their assigned units. This section covered their evaluation of both the introductory classes and the various team-leading responsibilities they had experienced. If their self-evaluations were considered satisfactory by supervisory personnel, they were transferred to their assigned units at the end of four weeks. The evaluation of each newcomer, along with that of the inservice coordinator, was given to the head nurse on the assigned unit so

that this administrator might gain insight into the ongoing practice needs of the new members of her staff.

The new graduates remained on the day shift of their permanent units from one to six weeks, depending on their adjustment to the new areas, and rotations to other shifts were scheduled with those of experienced graduates. The last portion of the evaluation form, designed to elicit their opinions of the total orientation period (Figure 3), was to be completed by the new nurses after four weeks on their assigned units.

Results of the Orientation Unit

Most of the new graduates placed on the orientation unit were transferred to their permanently assigned areas in four weeks and adjusted well. Feedback from the 1973 summer orientation program revealed that new graduates were pleased with their introduction to the hospital. Two areas of concern, however, were noted. First, in the opinion of some of the nurses, not enough experience had been given in the transcription of doctors' orders; and second, separation pains developed when these nurses were transferred from one unit to another. Most of them indicated, however, that this experience was short-lived and that they were accepted into their permanent units rather smoothly.

One graduate was kept on the orientation unit for an additional four weeks because the prospective head nurse was on vacation. Another was kept on the unit to provide more guidance in team leading, since her diploma program had not provided education or experience in team nursing. Two graduates were reassigned by joint agreement of the assistant director and inservice coordinator because of anticipated conflicts with the head nurse.

Since the advent of the orientation unit in May, 1973, 25 new graduates from the three types of nursing schools, with the exception of our own nursing program, have gone through the orientation program as described. Attrition from May to November has been limited to only one graduate, who had transportation difficulties. During 1972 we employed 24 new graduates, and the attrition rate from May through November was 7.5.

Evaluation of the program by means of a questionnaire for the head nurses also showed an acceptance of this new approach. These head nurses indicated that new graduates coming from the orientation unit were more confident than nonparticipants in their use of care plans, administration of medications, transcription of orders, use of departmental services, and making assignments, and that these new nurses were generally more competent in assuming team-leading responsibilities. They recommended that all newly employed graduates be placed on the orientation unit to provide a more rounded experience for these new personnel. Only two out of the 11 medical and surgical head nurses said they would rather orient their new graduates themselves.

The inservice coordinators have very positive feelings

regarding this approach to orientation, which provides a workable way for us to guide new employees into the work environment. Through close observation and assessment of the new graduate nurse, evaluations have not only more accurately provided for new graduates' needs, but also have helped us to meet nursing service requirements. We also found that the orientation unit allowed new graduates to learn together, eliminating the isolated feeling that sometimes occurs when an inexperienced graduate is placed in a new environment with experienced nurses.

Although the orientation unit has proved successful in our organization, we do not advocate the removal of the head nurse as a role model and developer for the new member of his or her staff. In many working situations it becomes difficult for a head nurse to devote the time needed to develop a new graduate, and the inservice coordinator serves as partner to the head nurse in this function. The inservice coordinator is able to provide a new staff member with basic nursing skills—knowledge of specific hospital policy for the administration of medications, transcription of doctors' orders, and an exposure to team-leading responsibilities, skills that develop confidence and that stimulate the new graduate to assume more patient and nursing staff teaching. There has also been an assessment made of the new graduate's abilities and limitations that should serve as a guideline for the head nurse in planning further development of the new member of the staff. If the inservice coordinator is able to provide a firmer foundation for the new

FIGURE 3. **Thomas Jefferson University Hospital Nursing Service**
evaluation of registered nurse orientation

(To be completed after four weeks on Permanent Unit)

Please answer the following questions. If you mark "sometimes," please explain on the back of this page.

	Yes	No	Some-times
1. I found that my questions were readily answered by personnel.	____	____	____
2. I found the orientation time moving too slowly.	____	____	____
3. The Inservice Coordinator assisted me in my adjustment to the unit.	____	____	____
4. I was given enough time and explanations to learn "routines" before starting P.M.'s or Nights.	____	____	____
5. The Head Nurse participated in my orientation.	____	____	____
6. I feel that I am part of the team.	____	____	____
7. My introduction and supervision of the medication system were satisfactory.	____	____	____
8. I found the progression of Team Member, Team Leader, and introduction to charge responsibilities helpful to my growth on the unit.	____	____	____
9. I feel comfortable with most of the nursing procedures performed on my unit.	____	____	____
10. I was made to feel welcome at Jefferson.	____	____	____
11. My team leading experience here at Jefferson was beneficial.	____	____	____
12. More follow-up by the Inservice Coordinator should have been carried out.	____	____	____
13. I feel that I needed additional time for the Head Nurse to explain and demonstrate problem-solving techniques.	____	____	____
14. I found it difficult to move from the orientation unit to my permanently assigned patient care area.			
Who appeared to be your best source for the questions you had?	____	____	____

_____

Discuss briefly any suggestions or comments you may have regarding your orientation time.

Inservice Coordinator's Comments:

graduate, the task of the preliminary development of the new nurse is made easier, and the head nurse can then begin to integrate further the new graduate's nursing education into the working situation.

To continue the stimulation of further nursing growth and leadership, three months after most of the new graduates had been at the hospital, the inservice coordinators planned and conducted a workshop. The new graduates had been in the working environment long enough to have gained some first-hand experience in providing patient care and in performing as team leaders. This workshop was designed to bring all the newly employed graduates together to discuss their nursing activities and frustrations. Topics chosen for the all-day conference included (1) adapting into a new role—reality vs. theory; (2) guides for leadership—the head nurse, supervisor, and assistant director; (3) communication tools for action; and (4) how to work through others for change.

As for any new program, adjustments still must be made in our project. At one point we had a large number of new personnel arriving, a situation that proved awkward in providing continuity of experiences. Our new nursing employees begin at the start of our biweekly pay period, and at present no control has been put on the size of the employee group that may enter at any one time. We found that when formal orientation classes exceeded 12 new graduates, the size of the group did not allow the openness that stimulates questions of the speakers normally experienced by the central orientation division. On the orientation unit, the inservice coordinator found it difficult to give individualized attention to the new graduate's practice needs, provide for meaningful experiences, and increase their nursing responsibilities, when 10 or more new employees were present.

Critics of an orientation unit concept voice a major concern over the anxiety that new graduates will experience when they are taken from one patient care area to another in a short period of time. The new graduates' evaluations of the program indicated that this did not seem to be a major difficulty; any uneasiness was short-lived at worst. Several new graduates stated that they were used to moving from one hospital to another for their student nursing experiences; consequently, moving from one patient care area to another in the same hospital did not prove threatening.

After evaluating the head nurses' recommendation that the program be extended to all graduates employed, we reviewed our decision not to include graduates from our own schools and realized that perhaps we had done them an injustice. Even though these new graduates may be familiar with hospital policies and procedures, they still need assistance in moving from the dependent student role to independent graduate responsibilities.

Modifications of the orientation unit concept have also proved to be of assistance to the 34 other new nursing employees who have come to work in the hospital's medical and surgical units since May, 1974. These include 25 experienced registered nurses, 12 new graduate practical nurses, and 9 experienced licensed practical nurses. Each new nurse brings to the employing institution a varying amount of nursing experience. Consequently each new employee was asked to fill out the three-section questionnaire. The skills inventory section was instrumental in acquainting the inservice coordinator with the number of nursing procedures the experienced graduates were competent in performing. The length of time spent on the orientation unit for these experienced newcomers depended on their previous nursing experience, their adaptation to delivery of patient care at the hospital, and their performance of team-leading responsibilities. These newcomers also were required to attend all the general introduction classes given by the central orientation division to acquaint them with hospital services.

The differences in preparation and competence among nursing practitioners prepared by nursing educational institutions has created a state of affairs within the work setting for which it has been difficult in the past for nursing services administrators to plan. New graduates come to the hospital with a significant amount of nursing theory and little clinical nursing experience. The nursing service administration at Thomas Jefferson University Hospital decided that an individualized orientation program on a selected patient care area would serve to offset the frustration and trauma of the beginning practitioner of nursing, while at the same time fulfilling the needs of the hospital within a reasonable time frame.

On the orientation unit, meaningful clinical experiences were planned after assessing the new graduates' nursing education, skills inventory, and work performance. This provided the beginning practitioners with some practical knowledge of delivering patient care on an independent level along with the awareness of team-leading responsibilities. The head nurses have found the new graduates more confident in planning patient care; the inservice coordinators have found that after the introductory orientation contact the rapport needed to plan progressive nursing leadership and assessment skills through education is present; and finally, the graduates themselves have felt more comfortable in the work environment after this adjustment period. Our experience with the orientation unit has enabled us to alleviate anxiety within the new graduate, therefore bridging the gap from the student role to the beginning practitioner role.

REFERENCES

1. Del Bueno, D. J., Quaifi, M., White, C. Grouping newcomers on an orientation unit. *American Journal of Nursing* 70:295–296, 1970.
2. Dennen, C. An orientation–rotation program for newly graduated nurses. *The Journal of Continuing Education in Nursing* 3:8–9, 1972.
3. Hahn, M. and Magill, K. A bridge over troubled waters. *The Journal of Continuing Education in Nursing* 4:15–19, 1973.
4. Mackety, C. K. Orientation program for the new O.R. nurse. *AORN Journal* 17:88–90, 1973.

PATIENT CARE CONFERENCES:

An Opportunity for Meeting Staff Needs

by Mary Ellen Palmer

Adapted from a "live" nursing care conference conducted on one of the nursing units at the Medical Center Hospital of Vermont, this article illustrates how staff needs can be met through a well-conducted patient care conference. The words used by the various workers to express thoughts are typical of their frame of reference and level of understanding. No attempt has been made to orient this presentation toward new theoretical content about cerebral vascular accidents.

Mary Ellen Palmer, R.N., M.S., is Associate Professor, School of Nursing, University of Vermont, Burlington, Vermont. This article is reprinted from JONA, March/April 1973.

To write about patient care conferences is commonplace; no one denies that such conferences provide the potential for delivering unified, consistent nursing care. This well-publicized purpose, however, can be expanded to include one other benefit, that of meeting staff needs for work satisfaction, personal recognition, and self-growth.

Picture the following situation: Three staff personnel—an R.N., a P.N., and a nurses' aide—about to have a twelve- to fifteen-minute conference concerning Mr. Johnson, a patient on their nursing unit. It may be assumed that this staff knew the following facts about Mr. Johnson and that they were well aware of his present status.

Mr. G. Johnson, seventy-five-years old, was admitted to the hospital on an emergency basis, accompanied by his wife. His admission was precipitated by a gradual increase in abdominal pain associated with "constipation" over a two- to three-day interval. Routine blood work indicated a hematocrit of 39 and a white count of 20,000 per cubic millimeter. Admission blood pressure was 160/100. Six hours after admission, Mr. Johnson's pain became more acute; an exploratory laparotomy revealed a volvulus, which was surgically reduced. Mr. Johnson's postoperative course was normal until the morning of the third day, when he

expressed concern about a "heavy feeling" in his left arm and leg. He also exhibited a slight slurring of speech. All of these symptoms became progressively worse, and by late afternoon a tentative diagnosis of cerebral thrombosis was noted on the clinical record.

The staff at this conference should be described briefly so that their particular personal needs will be recognizable. Miss R.N. is a friendly, approachable, highly experienced staff nurse. Miss P.N. is a young graduate of one month, enthusiastic, but inexperienced. Nurses' Aide, who has worked on this particular unit for five years, is a well meaning, middle-aged married woman who has "seen everything," so she says, and is willing to offer advice or opinions on practically any topic.

The conference proceeds as follows:

MISS R.N.: I thought Mr. Johnson would be appropriate to discuss today because of his most recent diagnosis. Here we were all ready to care for an uncomplicated surgical patient and now we have two sets of nursing concerns—that of a third-day, postoperative patient and that of a newly diagnosed, and hence possibly changing CVA patient. Maybe we could start by reviewing some of his current orders in the light of this latest problem. For example: bed rest. Dr. Andrews said Mr. Johnson would be on bed rest for the next 4 to 6 days to discourage further bleeding from his brain clot. I wonder what this implies from our viewpoint.

MISS P.N.: Well, I haven't taken care of many CVA patients, but I think that the present post-op orders should still be continued—I mean the deep breathing, and turning—just because he's still a surgical patient.

MISS R.N.: Yes, and those orders give us a good start on his CVA needs, too. His weakened left chest region adds to the need for the deep breathing, which is also the

49

reason for the CO_2 inhalation order for five minutes every hour. The frequent turning will be extremely important because of the decreased sensation on his left side. In fact, we should watch for even the slightest redness and not turn him on that side at all if this occurs; just use the right side and back and later the abdomen—as his operative side heals.

MISS P.N.: Shouldn't we give him special back care every time we turn him? He's so thin!

MRS. AIDE: Hmmm, I'd say we'd better do more skin care than just the back; but it doesn't really matter a lot of times what you do—they break down anyway.

MISS R.N.: Sometimes it is discouraging when we try so hard. However, you do have a good point about doing more than just the back—we must include massage of all bony prominences—heels, shoulder blades, elbows and buttocks, particularly on the left side. Now, another order is for "range of motion exercises to the affected side." This is clear enough, but let's not forget the unaffected side either. He can do this if we remind him to move his neck, right arm, and right leg; encourage him to turn himself on the right side by gripping the side rail; and have him use his right leg and arm to move his affected leg and arm. This will make him feel that he can do part of his care, and it will also remind him that the affected side is still a part of him—to be helped by other parts of him.

MISS P.N.: Gee, that sounds like a neat idea. I just thought of something else, though. Aren't there special ways to position these patients? I've never done it, but I remember seeing pictures of CVA patients with hand rolls, sand bags, and lots of pillows.

MISS R.N.: That's an excellent question. Yes, proper positioning will be extremely important for Mr. Johnson's future use of his affected arm and leg; and because the positioning is so specific, it will be easier to show than tell. So let's go in his room after this conference, and you can observe Mrs. Aide and me doing it.

MRS. AIDE: Okay, but I might as well tell you right now, Miss P.N., that the props never stay. You just turn around and pooh—you have to start all over again. It's an endless job!

MISS R.N.: It does seem to be quite often, especially when we get busy and time seems to fly. However, this just reminds us of the importance of checking the positioning aids whenever we are in the room—and that will be every hour for a while—with the CO_2 inhalations going on. Well, I wonder if there are any more things to discuss.

MISS P.N.: You mentioned earlier that his CVA picture could change. What things could happen to show this?

MISS R.N.: I'm glad you asked that. The same basic brain pathology which produced one clot could cause another, hence we should be particularly alert to changes in vital signs (he has them ordered for every 2 hours), changes in his ability to move or feel, changes in mood, and changes in degree of consciousness.

MRS. AIDE: Well, I sure hope I can make out his speech. Nothing is more annoying than when they can't make you understand what they want.

MISS R.N.: Yes, this certainly makes us feel helpless. Sometimes when I get in this spot, I say, "I know you must feel bad when you try so hard and we still don't understand you." Then, I either suggest to the patient that he try again; or if he acts very frustrated, that he stop for now and try again later. It will be very important for Mr. Johnson's self-concept that we praise him when he does communicate effectively and make every effort to make him feel worthy and useful in other ways—such as referring in positive tones to his normal side and encouraging him to do all he can for himself, including partial bathing and self-feeding.

MISS P.N.: Maybe we could ask his wife to also help us by letting him do things for himself. I've noticed she tends to wait on him.

MISS R.N.: Yes, we must try to get to know her almost as well as Mr. Johnson because his continued progress at home will depend more on her than on us. Maybe for a few days we could give her a chance to express how she feels about this new setback, and then we can evaluate better just how much she will be able to carry on in the same way that we do. This time will also give us the chance to observe Mr. Johnson's relationship with her and his attitude about his change of condition, so we can decide whether they both will fight to "get up or give up," so to speak. I wonder if there are any more questions. If not, let's try some of your good ideas and talk about our progress with Mr. Johnson again soon.

It should be noted that the above patient care conference was carefully planned and implemented so that it met several criteria: It was focused on one patient's personalized needs for unified, consistent care and emphasized the current nursing concerns of the patient. Such a conference is not the proper place for an overview of all future possibilities for the person, nor for an extensive review of such cardboard knowledge as pathology, medical therapy, and diagnostic tests.

The conference was limited to less than fifteen minutes, which is practical for a busy nursing service unit. It was conducted in such a way that the expression of facts, opinions, and attitudes were accepted without ridicule, censure, or disapproval. Nonmedical terminology was used so that Mrs. Nurses' Aide could understand—for example, the term *brain clot* was used rather than the term *intracranial lesion*; *speech loss* rather than *expressive aphasia*, and skin care to *shoulder blades* rather than to the *scapulae*. The staff were able to leave the conference with the feeling that there were some definite common goals to work toward with (not *for* or *on*) Mr. Johnson and his wife. Also, the door was left open for further staff planning as a group for continued care, as his needs changed.

During this patient care conference, staff members presented a variety of needs—needs for factual information, for reassurance, for technique demonstration, and for the chance to vent feelings of frustration and futility. As a result of this conference, staff members could be helped to achieve further self-growth via the assistance of Miss R.N., as is portrayed in the following vis-a-vis exchanges. In each of the following situations, assume that (1) Miss R.N. actually observed the incidents being discussed and that (2) these exchanges were held in privacy. Also, note that all of these learning sessions have as their starting focus some reference to Mr. Johnson and his care.

The first communication is between Miss R.N. and Miss P.N.

MISS R.N.: I wonder how you feel now about caring for Mr. Johnson. I remember you said at our conference a few days ago that you hadn't cared for too many CVA patients.

MISS P.N.: Oh, I felt much better after the conference; and I enjoy being assigned to him. However, I still feel kind of uncomfortable talking to him. I'm never sure· I say the right things—especially now, when he acts so depressed. In a way, it seemed much easier when he couldn't talk.

MISS R.N.: It's not easy to work with an attitude of pessimism, especially when you really want the person to get better—why, the way I see you go—if your enthusiasm and willpower could do it alone, I'm sure he would have been home long before this.

MISS P.N.: I try so hard. What else can I do?

MISS R.N.: Nothing for now. Somehow, he has to want to do it, and it's really too early to tell whether he will be motivated or not. However, this unhappy phase is a normal one and, while he's in it, we have to slow our pace to his and try to encourage him to express how he feels. For example, the other day, I heard him say to you, "I'll probably never get out of this bed." Now, what do you think he was really saying?

MISS P.N.: Oh, I remember that! And I said, "Of course you'll get out of that bed, Mr. Johnson. Remember, you're going to PT for the first time today." I suppose he was really saying how discouraged he was feeling.

MISS R.N.: Yes, and I wondered what would have happened if you had said instead, "Gee, you sound quite upset, Mr. Johnson," or something to that effect.

MISS P.N.: Oh, I'm beginning to get the message. Here I was trying to cheer him up about getting out of bed and he probably didn't really mean that at all.

MISS R.N.: It's not easy to listen for feeling tones because it's so much a part of everyday conversation to respond to the factual statement. Also, to get more clues, observe his actions. Is he saying "Oh, I feel fine," but then acting apathetic, panicked, frightened, showing a low frustration level, and getting easily angry with staff?

MISS P.N.: Gee, I can hardly wait to try some other approaches. Thanks for helping me feel so much better!

The second communication, not necessarily on the same day, is between Miss R.N. and Mrs. Nurses' Aide.

MISS R.N.: I've noticed your special helpfulness to Miss P.N. She says you've shown her many valuable things in the care of Mr. Johnson.

MRS. AIDE: Well, there's no reason why I shouldn't help her. I've been here long enough, and heaven knows it's no fun caring for CVA patients. I don't see how she can stay so enthusiastic and eager.

MISS R.N.: Well, his care can be quite a challenge, and Miss P.N. is trying to meet this challenge. I've frequently noticed how patient you are with Mr. Johnson and how much he seems to respond to this.

MRS. AIDE: Well, I don't dislike him, you know. It's just that I don't like what a diagnosis of CVA means in general.

MISS R.N.: I'm glad your feelings about the diagnosis don't interfere with your liking him as a person. However, there is one thing about his care that I want to ask you about. I've noticed that you brush his teeth, dress him, feed him, and hand him things he can reach, even though he can do some aspects of these activities by himself. You probably have a reason for doing this.

MRS. AIDE: Yes, I feel sorry for him. It bothers me to see him struggle so. Also, it takes him too long to do these things. Why if I didn't dress him for PT, I'd be in his room twice as long as I am. And usually, I have plenty of other patients to do, you know!

MISS R.N.: I can see your reasons for this; however, the very heart of rehabilitation is self-sufficiency, and we must work to try to get Mr. Johnson to want to do for himself. Otherwise, even if we get him walking, where and what will he walk to?

MRS. AIDE: Well, I know that what you say is true, but I always feel "What's the use?" I keep remembering other patients with whom we've worked for months, gotten them completely well—and then what happens? Very soon they either return here with another CVA or you see in the paper that they've dropped dead at home. So, I say, "Why push them so much? Leave the poor souls alone to die in peace."

MISS R.N.: I'm sorry that all your past experiences with CVA patients have been so unrewarding. How would you like me to try to arrange with the VNA [Visiting Nurse Association] for you to visit a rehabilitated CVA patient at home so that you could see a positive situation? Also, your outlook might be brightened by the following facts: 90 percent of all CVA patients walk, and in a recent industrial study, it was found that 62 percent of CVA patients returned to work. An even more hopeful note for the future is that impending CVA symptoms can now be spotted up to a year ahead of the attack. Which means they [attacks] could even be prevented!

MRS. AIDE: I guess when you work in a hospital you see only the worst cases, and it's easy to believe that no one ever gets better. However, now that you mention the idea—Eisenhower had a CVA as well as a heart attack, didn't he?

MISS R.N.: Yes, and Walt Whitman had a CVA at age 39, but died at 73 of something else; and Pasteur had a CVA at age 45 and then worked for 27 years more.

MRS. AIDE: Well, this talk kind of helps—I'll try to remember it when I get discouraged over Mr. Johnson's care.

Certain characteristics of the above communicative exchanges made them particularly effective. They focused on a specific concern of the staff member which had been verbalized during the patient care conference. This approach tends to render the discussion less of a personal attack and more of a concern as to how staff can better care for Mr. Johnson. These vis-a-vis exchanges were limited to one or very few areas of concern, since more progress is possible if single items at a time are worked on, as compared to multiple items.

Only three to five minutes of time were involved, which is practical for a busy nursing service situation, and the dialogues were conducted in a manner to encourage staff members to express their ideas in a noncritical atmosphere. Note that Miss R.N. used conversation-encouraging phrases such as "I wonder how you feel . . . ," and "you probably have a reason for this," and that she tended to find praiseworthy areas to mention, prior to tactfully offering possible suggestions for improvement of care. Also, Miss R.N. obviously tried to encourage the staff members to arrive independently at their own solutions for each problem discussed.

It would seem, from the sample role play situations developed in this article, that brief and well-organized patient care conferences can meet the dual purpose of personalizing care as well as assisting the staff to grow in self-understanding. One might further theorize that the degree to which staff needs are met will in turn determine the degree to which various patient needs are recognized and treated.

Three related ideas might also be discussed in view of the successful goals which are possible to reach through the utilization of patient care conferences. If, for example, patient care conferences can take as simple a form as three staff members getting together for less than fifteen minutes, it should be possible to guarantee that all patients on the unit could be as well planned for as is Mr. Johnson. If one-to-one brief and incidental (not accidental) conferences are effective in changing the behavior of adult learners when approached via the route of a patient care conference, this method should be employed more consistently by the R.N.

The kinds of learning which can be derived from the use of the patient care conference makes this medium an excellent one for teaching staff how to participate in or conduct an effective conference as a way of providing leadership for patient care and a learned approach to nursing care. It thus would seem that meeting patient and staff needs are mutually interdependent, that both involve a "person-to-person" process which can be implemented through a systematic program of patient care conferences. As a matter of emphasis, it could be said that the strength of the patient care conference is the nurse and that the strength of the nurse is what results from the patient care conference.

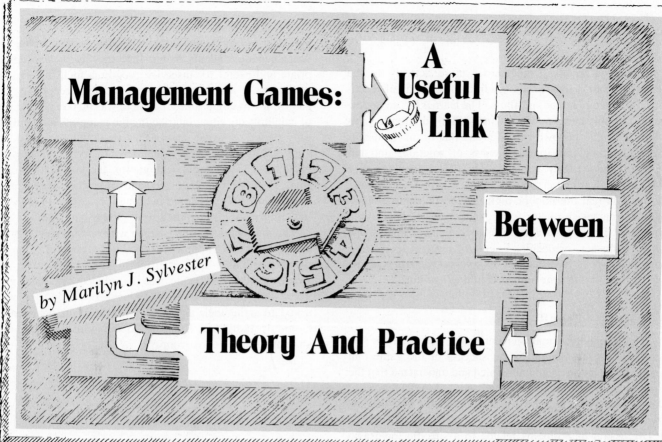

Management Games: A Useful Link Between Theory And Practice

by Marilyn J. Sylvester

The development of management skills is facilitated when the learner is actively involved in realistic nursing management situations. Simulation techniques are discussed as a way of providing realism and learner involvement problem-solving experiences in nursing management. These techniques can be used in inservice programs and university courses.

Major Marilyn J. Sylvester (Army Nurse Corps), B.S.N., M.N., is chief, Medical and Psychiatric Nursing Section, Madigan Army Medical Center, Tacoma, Washington. This article is reprinted from JONA, July-August, 1974.

Management theory, with its contributions from the behavioral scientists can, and frequently does, provide for a stimulating lecture or discussion on management techniques for nurses. Unfortunately, the desired results that effective managers of patient care seek will not automatically follow if the gap between theory and practice is not bridged.

Nurses involved in the management of patient care need depth in problem-solving and decision-making skills. Few inservice programs and university courses designed to develop nursing management skills provide realistic experiences that permit nurses to apply theoretical material in concrete nursing management situations. Simulation may be used to provide this type of learning experience.

Simulation techniques have been used in schools of business administration and management development programs as a link between theory and real life situations [1–3]. Parry describes these techniques as "situations that simulate the problems, constraints and resources of the everyday work environment. We then place the learner in the midst of the maze and ask him to find his way to the goal" [4]. Simulation techniques or management games include, among others, the case study method, in-basket exercises, and role play.

The *case study method* calls for the examination, analysis, and discussion of a particular management problem. *In-basket exercises* require the participants to assume the role of a manager and individually take action on several letters, papers, and memos in their incoming mail. Once the decisions are completed, the participants share their decisions and rationale. *Role play* involves two or more persons acting out the roles called for in a situation. The situation may be partially structured or completely spontaneous. Following the enactment, there is a discussion of the appropriateness of actions taken by the participants.

ADVANTAGE OF MANAGEMENT GAMES

Management games are particularly well suited to applying several management principles, namely, planning, organizing, coordinating, decision-making, and control. They provide valuable experience in problem-solving human relations situations that include communication, motivation, and leadership.

As a result of active participation and intense involvement by the student, learning usually takes place in three phases. The student learns the *facts* that are part of the game context and dynamics; the *processes* that are simulated by the game; and the advantages and disadvantages of *alternative decision-making strategies* [5].

Simulation *involves* the learner more actively in the learning process than do the traditional methods of teaching, i.e., lectures, reading, films. The learner has an opportunity to apply new knowledge and skill in addition to gaining insight into his own behavior and that of others. Feedback regarding the appropriateness of solutions and behavior is immediately available. Since the learner is active throughout, learning is more efficient. The price of a wrong decision in real life may be high, and participants in management games can learn from experience without paying this price. Broad generalizations are avoided as to how one *might* plan, act, or decide. Events of the real world that may take weeks to occur can be compressed into a single game, thus saving time and accelerating learning.

BEFORE AND AFTER THE GAME

Prior to playing a management game, the instructor sets the stage. It is essential to the success of the game that learners feel involved and motivated and understand that the game is relevant to their learning needs. Material related to the game may be presented in a lecture, or a film may be used.

Discussion of problems related to a specific topic also serves as an introduction to the particular game involved. For example, the instructor may give a lecture on factors to consider in making patient care assignments and follow the lecture with a game that calls for the application of principles presented in the lecture. The instructor might conclude his lecture by saying, "These are some important factors to keep in mind when making patient care assignments. Let's see how these points can be applied to a real life situation." The instructor may set the stage for a management game pertaining to employee motivation by asking, "Have you encountered problems with personnel who lack interest in their jobs?"

During the postgame discussions, learners and instructor share their feelings and the lessons learned in the application of concepts and skills. "Although it is nice to win games, it is in the analysis and discussion (rather than in the outcome per se) that most of the learning takes place. In this regard, everyone who plays the game is a winner" [6].

THE CLASSROOM EXPERIENCE

While concurrently supervising the team leadership experience and teaching the management theory course to senior baccalaureate nursing students at the University of Maryland, Walter Reed Army Institute of Nursing, the author observed that students often expressed difficulty in applying the nursing management theory to the team leadership experience. To facilitate application of the principles to realistic nursing management situations, several management games were designed by the author. Although these

games had been created for use in a management course for baccalaureate students in nursing, they were also appropriate and useful for inservice programs focusing on staff development and leadership training. Before playing the games, it was emphasized that there was no one correct way of handling any situation (playing the game); there would be only better or worse approaches or solutions. Also, the approach and its success would depend largely upon careful analysis of the situation (the game), the assets and limitations of the persons involved, and an attitude of receptiveness for necessary changes in thought or course of action as new information is acquired or as new events occur.

The management course began with an overview of management history and proceeded to a discussion of planning, problem-solving, and decision-making. Following the overview, the first game was introduced. Students were given the same Disaster Planning Exercise. They were asked to write their answers to the problem depicted by Game 1. Individual solutions to the problem were then shared with the entire group.

Game I. Disaster Planning.

There has been an earthquake. You have been assigned the responsibility of caring for fifty patients. There is no electricity or water supply. Your patients have the following types of injuries: burns, fractures, soft tissue wounds. Your "treatment facility" is a large room in a grade school. The following is a list of equipment and supplies that are available. No additional support will be available for five days. You may select seven items from this list. Which would you choose? Why?

Packaged food	IV solution
Flashlights	Injectable penicillin
Stethoscope	Drinking water
Oxygen tank	Sterile basins
Aspirin	Ambu bag
Sterile dressings	Blankets
Bandage scissors	

Table I shows the student selection of disaster care items before class discussion of the problem. During class discussion of the problem, several factors became apparent. First, in some cases the students had insufficient information to fully weigh all the alternatives. Did the flashlights have batteries? Would there be scissors at the school? Were needles and IV tubing included with the penicillin and IV solution? How could the oxygen be administered? Would the school have a food supply on hand? Second, most had not

Table I. NURSING CARE ITEMS SELECTED BEFORE DISCUSSION OF A DISASTER PLANNING GAME.

Item	N	%
Flashlights	26	100
Drinking water	26	100
Blankets	25	96
Food	24	92
Sterile dressings	21	80
Aspirin	18	70
IV solution	13	50
Injectable penicillin	11	42
Ambu bag	7	27
Scissors	6	23
Oxygen	5	19
Stethoscope	0	0
Sterile basins	0	0

explored all facets of the situation. Aspirin could be used for several purposes: reduce pain and temperature and provide some psychological support in that something is being done. Dressings could be used for splinting in addition to wound care. An IV solution could be used for drinking and/or cleansing wounds if not for IV therapy. Penicillin may not have needles included, and there would be no way of treating an unfavorable reaction to it. Probably other antibiotics would be available in five days. Mouth-to-mouth resuscitation could be used instead of the Ambu bag. Blankets would be needed to provide warmth and for splints.

Table II. CHANGES IN SELECTION OF NURSING CARE ITEMS AFTER DISCUSSION OF A DISASTER PLANNING GAME.

	N	%
No change	4	15
1 or 2 changes	22	85

Items rejected after discussion	Items selected after discussion
Oxygen	IV solution
Scissors	Sterile dressings
Ambu bag	Aspirin
Penicillin	Packaged food
	Drinking water
	Blankets

Table II shows changes in the selection of items after class discussion of the problem.

Significant experience was gained in problem-solving and decision-making as each individual scrutinized the items for potential use in the disaster situation. While working on the problem alone, and later in group discussion, the need for gathering pertinent information and exploring reasonable assumptions became evident. The fact that 85 percent of the group changed one or two choices following discussion of the problem further indicated the importance of using available resources and pooling knowledge in the decision-making process.

Planning a continuing education program was the subject of a game which emphasized decision-making and coordination. Using a schematic format adapted from PERT (Program Evaluation Review Technique) [7], students were directed to diagram the events in the sequence in which they thought they should occur. They were encouraged to explore all possible ways of arranging the events. Game 2 shows the events, each numbered for the purpose of diagraming. The most frequently selected sequences are represented in Figure I.

Game 2.

Continuing Education Planning Game Event

Number	Event
0	Start
1	Date, time, place established
2	Program announced
3	Speaker selected
4	Audience defined
5	Evaluation form answered
6	Topic selected
7	Program conducted
8	Objectives formulated
9	Evaluation form written

While equally valid arguments may be offered for the arrangement of some of the events, one fact stands out. Certain events must precede others: determination of date, time, and place must occur before the program is announced and conducted; the evaluation form must be written before it can be answered; objectives should be written before the evaluation form is tackled; and, finally, the program must be conducted prior to answering the evaluation form. Several questions were discussed: How can time be used most efficiently? Which sequence allows for the most flexibility?

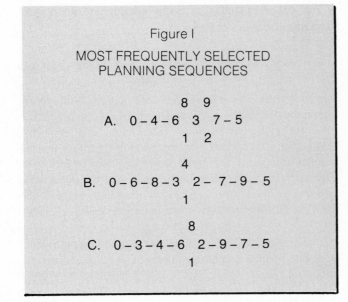

Figure I

MOST FREQUENTLY SELECTED
PLANNING SEQUENCES

```
            8  9
A.  0 – 4 – 6   3   7 – 5
            1  2

            4
B.  0 – 6 – 8 – 3   2 – 7 – 9 – 5
            1

            8
C.  0 – 3 – 4 – 6   2 – 9 – 7 – 5
            1
```

As the management course progressed, the process of organization was discussed. Types of authority and the concepts of delegation and decentralization were explored. Game 3 was used to apply this theoretical information.

Game 3. Delegating Authority

You are the assistant head nurse. Upon returning from lunch, you have been informed of the following matters that need your attention:

1. A visitor has fainted.
2. Mr. Smith's IV has infiltrated, and he is far behind on his fluids.
3. Four patients have not received their lunch trays. It is 1:00 P.M.
4. The operating room supervisor just called and said to give Mrs. Jones her pre-op Demerol now.
5. The toilet is overflowing in the patient's rest room. Water and feces are pouring out rapidly.

The following personnel are available. Who should do what and in which order of priority?

You (assistant head nurse), Unit Manger, Ward Clerk, and L.P.N.

After group discussion of this situation, most students agreed that the following would be the best solution: The assistant head nurse should attend first to the visitor who has fainted. The LPN discontinues Mr. Smith's IV, and the unit manager checks the flooded rest room. While all this is going on, the ward clerk calls the maintenance department for the plumber and the dietary service for the missing trays. Once the assistant head nurse determines that the visitor's condition is stable, she assigns the LPN to stay with the visitor. The assistant head nurse is then free to administer · the Demerol and restart the IV.

Two basic decisions are called for in this exercise. First, who is best qualified to handle each task and, second, what is the order of priority in handling them? Students rarely have difficulty with the former decision; however, they frequently feel they need more information to determine priorities. For example, they want to know how sick is Mr. Smith? Who said the visitor fainted? How soon will Mrs. Jones go to the OR? What is the physical arrangement of the ward?

It is interesting to note that when this game was first played, the item "a visitor has fainted" originally read "a student nurse has fainted." None of the students felt that caring for the student nurse should be the assistant head nurse's first priority. When questioned about this, they responded that the instructor would take care of the student. It was pointed out that the game did not include an instructor. To eliminate this element of overidentification, visitor was substituted for student nurse. This illustrates that unexpected outcomes may result in the actual playing of games. When undesired results occur, revisions must be made to provide the intended learning experience.

The remainder of the management course dealt with discussions on leadership, motivation, interpersonal relationships, personnel orientation, counseling, patient care assignments, and conferences. Several other management games were utilized to allow for supervised practice in applying management theory. The following is an example of one of them:

Miss Lewis is a licensed practical nurse who was assigned to your general surgical ward one month ago. She previously worked on a medical cardiac ward. Since her arrival, many patients have commented favorably about her concerned attitude. She is willing to help her coworkers and always completes her patient assignment on time. Ever since her arrival on your ward, she has taken 45 minutes for meals instead of the allotted 30 minutes. This has just recently been called to your attention by the 3 to 11 nurse with whom she works. Yesterday she was observed disposing of contaminated dressings in a patient's wastebasket instead of the designated area for disposal of contaminated materials. You have scheduled a counseling session with her for tomorrow. How would you handle these matters with her?

STUDENT REACTION TO GAMES

Student reaction to the management games was positive. At the end of each semester, the students were asked to complete a written anonymous critique of the management course. There was unanimous agreement that the most valuable aspect of the course was the simulation experience. Some typical comments made by students were: ''The games we played in class gave me more confidence in making decisions and handling personnel problems during my team leading experience.'' ''By all means continue the management games; in fact, it would be helpful to have more of them.'' ''It was very helpful to see how different people viewed the same situation. This increased my awareness of the need to thoroughly analyze problems.''

Several management games were played before the students participated in real life nursing management situations. They felt that the games enabled them to examine problems more closely and explore alternative courses of action. Classroom experience also demonstrated how prone they were to misdiagnose problems or fail to explore the ramifications of actions directed toward the solution of problems.

Skills were developed in human relations as the students examined different approaches to dealing with people. Feedback from the group discussion increased self-awareness and instilled confidence in their ability to handle similar situations in the clinical setting.

SUMMARY

Nurses in, or preparing for, management positions have a continuing need to develop their management skills. A realistic learning environment is valuable in programs designed to develop nursing management skills.

Lectures and reading assignments are important for imparting information. To be an effective manager, however, more than information is required. Skills must be learned to do the job, and they require experience. It is in the acquiring of experience that the teacher's role takes on a new perspective. He must provide the student with learning experiences designed to allow for the application of management concepts and skills. Management games provide this critical link between theory and practice.

REFERENCES

1. Kibbee, J. M., Craft, C. J., and Nanus, B. *Management Games, A New Technique For Executive Development.* New York: Reinhold Publishing Corp., 1961.
2. Greenlaw, P. S., Herron, L. W., and Rawdon, R. H. *Business Simulation in Industrial and University Education.* Englewood, N.J.: Prentice Hall, Inc., 1962.
3. Boocock, S. S., and Schild, E. O. *Simulation Games In Learning.* Beverly Hills, Calif.: Sage Publications, Inc., 1968.
4. Parry, S. B. The name of the game . . . is simulation. *Training Develop.* 25:28, 1971.
5. Boocock, S. S., and Schild, E. O. *Op. cit.*, p. 78.
6. Parry, S. B. *Op. cit.*, p. 32.
7. Richards, M. D., and Greenlaw, P. S. *Management Decision Making.* Homewood, Ill.: Richard D. Irwin, Inc., 1966, pp. 423–429.

SENSITIVITY TRAINING

by Rolf E. Rogers

Rolf E. Rogers, M.A., Ph.D., is professor of management and coordinator, Behavioral Science Group, University of Alberta, Edmonton, Canada. The author of three books and numerous articles and research monographs in organizational behavior and management theory, his current research in organizational and managerial stress has received international attention. This article is reprinted from JONA, November-December, 1972.

Dr. Rogers analyzes whether sensitivity training is an effective device for improving management effectiveness in formal organizations. The assumptions and modes of operation of a T (training)-group is established and compared to group psychotherapy. The author concludes that sensitivity training may be effective if a T-group is identified by a qualified consultant as the optimum solution to an organizational problem and if sufficient safeguards and control mechanisms are employed to protect the individual and the organization.

Sensitivity training, encounter groups, T-groups, the laboratory approach, and so forth, have invaded organizational life in recent years with their claim for increased management effectiveness through interpersonal relations. Increasing effectiveness in management and interpersonal interaction among members of formal organizations is a laudable goal. Our question is whether sensitivity training can achieve this goal and whether it is a desirable training device for formal organizations.

Caveat Emptor

THE T-GROUP

The T (training)-group is the most common type of sensitivity training used in a formal organization, the type of organization traditionally found in industry and the health sciences. Examples are manufacturing, sales and service organizations, hospitals, and medical clinics. This type of organization is essentially bureaucratic. To a greater or lesser degree, all bureaucratic organizations observe the imperatives of the Weberian model, namely (1) a clear division of labor, (2) a chain of command, (3) abstract procedures, (4) impersonal application of rules, and (5) technical qualification for all employees.[1] In short, a formal organization is designed on the basis of rationality, efficiency, and technological competence.

Into this setting of rationality and efficiency, the T-group is introduced to "sensitize" the organizational participants. The objective of the T-group, in this context, is to provide the maximum possible opportunity for participants to:

1. Expose their behavior
2. Give and receive feedback from the group
3. Experiment with new behavior
4. Develop awareness and acceptance of self and others.[2]

By design, the interaction of participants in a T-group is unstructured. There is no agenda, there are no specific norms of group behavior, and there is no leader, except for a trainer in some groups.

According to Argyris,[3] the desirable sequence of events in a T-group begins with a *dilemma*—when habitual actions are not effective; second, *inventive action*—the exploration of new ways and the heightening of "diagnostic" skills; third, *unfreezing*—where old behavior is being abandoned but new behavior is not yet invented; fourth, *learning through feedback*—participants react in the dilemma—invention situation in the group; and fifth, *generalizing*—to what extent does laboratory behavior fit outside (real world) situations.

In sensitivity training the assumption is made that the participants are "normal." However, there are no preliminary testing or diagnostic interviews to determine normalcy. In addition, T-group participation in a formal organization is allegedly voluntary. Is it voluntary when the "boss" calls in his junior manager and tells him: "Joe (or Mary), I have recommended you for a T-group session at Beaver Lake this weekend. Of course, you don't have to go, if you don't want to. I can send George (or Josephine), but I thought you should have the first chance"? This is hardly voluntary. If Joe (or Mary) refuses, the boss might wonder "What's wrong with him—does he have something to hide—maybe he is not 'good' management material after all."

T-GROUP VS. GROUP PSYCHOTHERAPY

The underlying assumptions of a T-group may be compared with those prevalent in traditional group psychotherapy. The reason for using group psychotherapy for this purpose is the mounting concern that sensitivity training, in varying degrees: (1) induces stress, (2) deals with the unconscious motivations of participants, (3) uses clinical constructs and methodology, and (4) focuses on personal past history. These four imperatives are basic elements in group psychotherapy. In other words, the more a T-group deals with and becomes involved in these imperatives, the more it is group psychotherapy.

The purpose of group psychotherapy is essentially the same as individual therapy, except that it is performed in a group setting. According to Foulknes and Anthony, "the emphasis in group psychotherapy is on the individual (in the group). Group dynamics exist, but have no bearing on the ongoing analysis, group or no group."[4] Group psychotherapy, therefore, employs controlled observation and guidance by a qualified analyst as opposed to the no leader-no control concept employed in a T-group.

Table 1 presents a comparison between T-group training and group psychotherapy.

Criterion 1. Are participants normal?

A T-group is supposed to deal with persons who do not manifest overt psychological problems or disturbances. This is obviously not the case in group psychotherapy. In the latter situation, patients are selected carefully for group therapy on the basis of their particular disorder and the probability of successful treatment in a group environment. However, since criterion 2 (Testing) is not used for a T-group, how do we know whether an individual has

TABLE 1

COMPARISON BETWEEN T-GROUP AND GROUP THERAPY

Underlying Criteria	T-Group	Group Therapy
1. Are participants normal?	Yes	No
2. Is preliminary testing and diagnosis used?	No	Yes
3. Is the group supervised by a qualified analyst during interaction?	No	Yes
4. Is the end-objective of the group interaction clearly defined and established?	No	Yes
5. Can the success of the group session(s) be measured?	No	Yes

TABLE 2

COMPARISON OF GROUP OPERATION BETWEEN T-GROUP AND THERAPY GROUP

Variables of Group Operation	T-Group	Group Therapy
1. Is there an agenda or established *modus operandi*?	No	Yes
2. Is the group environment threatening?	Yes	Yes
3. Is the interaction controlled by an expert?	No	Yes
4. Is clinical observation used?	No	Yes

psychological problems or not? Overt manifestation is not always associated with a psychological problem, nor does the average manager or trainer have the qualifications necessary to make such a determination. In short, the assumption that participants are normal is not only unrealistic but untenable, unless preliminary diagnostic techniques are employed.

Criterion 2. Preliminary testing and diagnosis

In group psychotherapy the diagnostic criteria used are as comprehensive as those used in individual therapy. Groups are carefully constructed and continual observation is exercised. There is no preliminary diagnosis in a T-group to determine whether participants are "normal" or suffering from neurotic or psychotic disturbances. The American Psychiatric Association, in a recent Task Force Report, noted that many of the encounter groups "recruit participants by word of mouth or written advertisement. Some teachers lead encounter groups in the classroom, housewives lead groups at their homes for their friends...."[5] In short, how can one assume that participants are normal without appropriate diagnosis and testing? And further, as a result of the induced stress of a T-group session, what is the potential damage to an individual who is "not normal?"

Criterion 3. Is the group supervised by a qualified analyst during interaction?

By qualified analyst we mean a psychiatrist or clinical psychologist. We do not consider an individual who has spent a few weeks in a "trainer" course qualified to assess stress manifestations and regressive tendencies in individual participants. In group psychotherapy, an individual who exhibits dysfunctional symptoms is removed from the group environment and his case is reassessed. Who will identify the stress manifestations of a participant in a T-group? Who will remove him from the group before it is too late? The average T-group does not have a qualified analyst, and even if one is present he does not have a diagnosis and history of each individual as does the analyst in the psychotherapy group.

Criterion 4. Is the end-objective of the group interaction clearly defined and established?

The answer in group psychotherapy is clear. The objective is treatment and solution of the psychological disturbance. What is the objective in a T-group? "Improving interpersonal relations," according to Argyris.[6] What does that mean? What standards are used? How is it measured? (See criterion 5.)

Criterion 5. Can the success of the group session(s) be measured?

This is dependent upon criterion 4. In order to measure anything, there must be a standard against which measurement can be made. In order to set a standard, there must be a clearly defined objective. In group psychotherapy, the patient either improves, regresses, or remains unchanged. The standard in this case is his behavior pattern at the time therapy commences. Continual measurement takes place during each session, and his actions are recorded as in individual therapy. Where is the standard in a T-group? There is no measurable objective, there are no records of the existing behavior patterns of the participants, there is no continual series of sessions (most T-groups are a one-time proposition), and who would perform the measurement—since there is no qualified analyst present?

Table 2 presents the second basis of comparison between T-groups and psychotherapy groups. The comparison base is the operation of the group during the actual sessions.

Variable 1. Is there an agenda or established modus operandi?

As noted earlier, a T-group does not, by design, use an agenda. The idea is that interaction should develop freely between participants. Therapy groups, on the other hand, have a *modus operandi* which is designed to achieve the maximum therapeutic benefit for each patient. The effect of no agenda in a T-group is increased stress, increased anxiety levels, and possible dysfunctional consequences to individual participants.

Variable 2. Is the group environment threatening?

The answer is "yes" in both groups. Any form of laboratory is, at best, an approximation of reality, but never reality itself. The T-group weekend at Beaver Lake is not representative of the home offices of the ABC Corporation or the wards and operating rooms of the XYZ Hospital. The deliberate relaxation of daily routine and bureaucratic imperatives represents a withdrawal from the real world. Any environmental change, especially one in which certain expectations are prevalent, causes increases in stress and anxiety manifested by frustration, aggression, or apathy. The expectations from a T-group session are to increase "interpersonal competence." There is the implicit expectation by the organization which is sending the individual to the session, and which is paying for it, to see a reasonable return for its investment. But how is this return measured? There is no empiric evidence that T-group training effects any significant change in overt behavior on the job.[7]

Variables 3 and 4. Is the interaction controlled by an expert and is clinical observation used?

Variables 3 and 4 are interrelated. A T-group is not, as a rule, supervised by a qualified analyst. Therefore, interaction is not controlled and clincial observation of participants does not exist. This control and observation is present in a psychotherapy group in which interaction is clinically controlled in relation to the type of interaction and its effect on each participant.

CAVEAT EMPTOR

What have been the effects of T-group training for organizations and individuals?

Effect on Organizations

There is no research evidence that sensitivity training changes behavior. Bass notes that "Whether sensitivity training increases sensitivity on the job or success as a leader on the job still has to be demonstrated."[8] Calame states that a growing number of companies "are taking a much more critical look at sensitivity training. . . . Many have modified their sensitivity programs to produce more company and job-oriented discussions and less probing into personal feelings and behavior. Others have dropped sensitivity training altogether."[9]

Aside from the inability of behavioral scientists to provide empiric evidence on the effects of sensitivity training in organizations, many companies today are looking closely at the cost-benefits ratio of sensitivity training; in other words, what are the financial benefits resulting from the cost of the training? What is the return on investment? Without empiric evidence, who knows?

There are valid reasons why empiric evidence is difficult to obtain. First, T-groups are generally one-time episodes; they do not have the continuity and observation time dimension required for empiric research. Second, participants return to an unchanged environment after the T-group experience. This introduces the so-called fading effect. What this means, simply, is that unless a certain type of behavior is reinforced by the organization and is consistent with organizational philosophy, that new behavior will create stress, anxiety, and frustration and will eventually be discontinued in favor of more traditional behavior. In other words, the T-group participant will revert to his former behavior because it is more acceptable to the organization. Third, in order to measure changes in behavior on the job resulting from sensitivity training, it would be necessary to observe pre- and post-training behavior in experimental and control groups. This latter

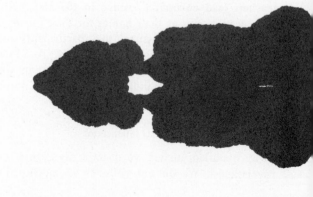

aspect is a complex research proposition. It has not been capable of successful application in establishing scientifically supportable findings. In short, the nature of sensitivity training is such that it has been impossible to establish scientifically sound research evidence supporting the benefit of sensitivity training for formal organizations. Without such evidence, cost-benefit analysis is not possible, nor, indeed are most other justifications for using T-group training as an agent in improving organizational effectiveness.

Effect on the Individual

The data relating to T-group casualties are extraordinarily difficult to evaluate. There are several reasons for this. First, the correlation between the T-group experience and subsequent psychological disturbances is virtually impossible to determine because there is no centralized agency or mechanism to collect, interpret, and report such occurrences. For example, if five of fifteen T-group participants develop psychological problems *after* the experience (anywhere from ten days to six months) and consult their own analyst, how can these problems be correlated with the specific T-group experience on a collective basis? Second, since a T-group has no "clinical control," how is it possible to identify the beginning manifestations of such problems as anxiety, depression, agitation, and psychotic reactions?

The majority of data available are, in general, limited to events occurring during the sessions and measured in terms of hospitalization, overt psychosis, or immediate need for psychiatric attention. Nevertheless, the Task Force Report of the American Psychiatric Association[10] contains a considerable number of reports in which "psychiatric casualties" are enumerated, for example:

- In one National Training Laboratory lab, 10 to 15 percent of the participants consulted the lab psychiatrist for such complaints as anxiety, depression, agitation and insomnia.
- In four two-week laboratories of 400 participants, 6

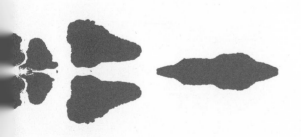

developed acute psychotic reactions.

- In three T-groups (a total of 32 participants), there was one psychotic reaction; one borderline acute psychotic withdrawal reaction; four marked withdrawal reactions with lack of participation in the group; two severe emotional breakdowns with acute anxiety, crying, and temporary departure from the group; one sadistic and exhibitionistic behavior pattern; and four mild anxiety or depressive reactions.
- In a T-group for psychiatric residents at the Menninger School of Psychiatry, out of 11 participants, 3 suffered psychotic breakdowns, two during the course of the meetings and one seven months after the meetings terminated.

The Committee on Mental Health of the Michigan State Medical Society recently conducted a study on sensitivity training laboratories in Michigan because of reports of psychotic breakdowns, exacerbation of preexisting marital difficulties, and an increase in life tensions.[10] The study committee concluded that the hazards were so considerable that all group leaders should be professional experts trained in the fields of mental illness and mental health.[11]

We must note, however, that although there are obvious dangers in the T-group experience, it is difficult to generalize. There is little question that group experience can be dangerous for some participants: "The more powerful the emotions evoked, the less clinically perspicacious and responsible the leader, the more psychologically troubled the group member, then the greater the risk of adverse outcome."[12]

CONCLUSIONS

Even though this paper is an implicit criticism of sensitivity training, sensitivity training per se in a normal organization is to be recommended, provided certain conditions are observed.

- Sensitivity training (T-group) appears to be the optimum solution to a specific organizational behavior problem. This means that a qualified management consultant has performed a diagnostic analysis of the organization, has identified the problem and its causes, has evaluated alternative solutions, and has decided that sensitivity training appears to be the optimum solution for this particular problem and this particular organization.
- A qualified analyst (psychiatrist or clinical psychologist) is employed to conduct T-group sessions.
- Preliminary testing and diagnosis is performed by the analyst on each scheduled participant. Those who are not suitable for sensitivity training are not permitted to participate (this preliminary interview should be treated as privileged information between analyst and employee).
- Participation in the T-group is strictly voluntary,

without explicit or implicit sanctions against any individual.

• The T-group session is observed and controlled by the analyst. Any participant exhibiting psychological dysfunctions is immediately removed from the group.

• The session should be oriented more toward a problem-solving type of interaction and should minimize the traditional emphasis on personal aspects of interaction. This criterion is implicit in our first condition. Since a specific problem (or problems) has been identified, the group should concentrate on the solution of this problem rather than on such ambiguities as "improvement of interpersonal relations."

• There should be some postsession observation period by the analyst to assure that at a later date, no dysfunctional psychological consequences arise in any of the participants.

• There should be a follow-up study by the management consultant to determine whether this approach was successful in solving the organization's problem.

In summary, sensitivity training in a formal organization is to be endorsed only *if* these safeguards are observed to protect the individual and the organization from unqualified and incompetent consultants and sensitivity training solicitors. If these safeguards are not employed then caveat emptor.

REFERENCES

1. Rogers, R. E. *The Political Process in Modern Organizations*, New York: Exposition Press, 1971, p. 141.
2. Argyris, C. T-groups for Organizational Effectiveness, *Harvard Business Review* 42 (2): 60-74, 1964.
3. Argyris, *op. cit.,* p. 61.
4. Foulknes, S. H., and Anthony, E. J. *Group Psychotherapy,* Baltimore: Penguin Books, 1965, p. 18.
5. American Psychiatric Association, *Encounter Groups and Psychiatry,* April, 1970, p. 5. Task Force Report.
6. Argyris, *op. cit.,* p. 63.
7. See for example the research by C. L. Cooper and I. L. Mangham, *T-groups: A Survey of Research,* New York: John Wiley and Sons, 1971, and G. S. Odiorne, The Trouble with Sensitivity Training, *Training and Development Journal* 17(10): 9, 1963.
8. Bass, B. Review of Leadership and Organization. *Journal of Business* 35 (3): 325, 1962. For additional evidence, see R. J. House, T-group Education and Leadership Effectiveness. *Personnel Psychology* 20 (1): 1, 1967.
9. Calame, B. E. The Truth Hurts. *The Wall Street Journal,* July 14, 1969, p. 1.
10. American Psychiatric Association, *op. cit.,* pp. 13-14.
11. American Psychiatric Association, *op. cit.,* p. 14.
12. American Psychiatric Association, *op. cit.,* p. 17.

Leadership Development at the Clinical Unit Level

Judy S. Wengerd
May L. Wykle
Helen M. Tobin

Workshops and individual guidance are two methods used to develop the leadership potential of registered nurses assigned to patient care units. The content for leadership development is based on the role expectations and therefore differs for the several groups of registered nurses from different basic educational programs. Content and reference building, teaching methods, and utilization of resource persons are discussed.

Judy Swope Wengerd, R.N., B.S.N., was instructor in staff development at University Hospitals of Cleveland and coordinator of leadership development programs for registered nurses at the time this article was written.

May Hinton Wykle, R.N., M.S.N., is assistant professor, psychiatric nursing, Frances Payne Bolton School of Nursing, Case Western Reserve University and works with senior students in their leadership experience. At the time this article was written, Mrs. Wykle served as a psychiatric nurse integrator at University Hospitals of Cleveland.

Helen M. Tobin, R.N., M.S.N., is director of centralized staff development, University Hospitals of Cleveland and associate clinical professor, Frances Payne Bolton School of Nursing, Case Western Reserve University. This article is reprinted from JONA, September-October, 1974.

Descriptions of leadership programs most frequently concentrate on leadership development of supervisory personnel. Equally pertinent, but often given little attention, is a program of leadership development for registered nurses assigned to patient care units.

In our setting, the organization of nursing is based on the concept of support rather than on control of organizational members in the traditional manner. Our philosophy of nursing regards recognition and reward for competent performance as well as opportunities for learning and advancement as vital forces in implementing the philosophy of the institution. The emphasis is not only on providing learning opportunities for all personnel but also that all personnel take advantage of these opportunities to the fullest extent possible. Concepts basic to effectively implementing these beliefs are planned change, decentralized decision-making, and an exemplary learning climate [1]. These factors have influenced the direction taken in providing for leadership development of registered nurses assigned to the patient care unit level. Both centralized and decentralized staff development activities are used in implementing the program.

Workshop and individual guidance are means used to develop leadership potential. Workshop content is based on separate role expectations for registered nurses with different educational preparation. Graduates of each group (associate degree, diploma, and baccalaureate degree programs) have unique learning needs. These learning needs are jointly identified by the workshop participants, the senior clinical nurses (head nurses) and assistant directors, and the centralized staff development instructors, and are used as guidelines for workshop content. In addition, responsibility for identifying and seeking learning opportunities is perceived as a responsibility of each individual staff member and is so stated in the role expectations for all categories of personnel [2].

CENTRALIZED STAFF DEVELOPMENT WORKSHOPS

Preparation for Centralized Workshops

Groundwork for leadership development is begun during the initial orientation period when classes are held on the philosophy and objectives of the nursing department, role expectations for self and others, select policies and procedures of the institution, and health care resources available to personnel and patients. During the first three to six months of their employment, new staff are provided decentralized clinical experiences focused on the roles of practitioner and beginning team leader. The senior clinical nurse is responsible for planning these experiences with the new staff member. Decentralized staff development continues in the clinical area on a continuous basis to help the staff member give comprehensive nursing care to a particular patient population.

Types of Centralized Workshops

Leadership development workshops are divided into three categories: basic, promotional, and continued. The basic workshop is designed to meet the needs of the new

employee and is offered following the initial three to eight months of employment. Because a system for promotion is available to the registered nurse staff, promotional workshops for meeting new or expanded roles are also offered.

Continued workshops are usually offered to groups of nurses who share similar role expectations and who have been in those positions for a period of time; for example, the senior clinical nurse role. One-day centralized workshops supplement the continuous decentralized leadership development provided by the director and assistant director of a clinical speciality.

Because most of our new registered nurse staff are recent graduates, the basic workshops prove suitable to their learning needs. Consideration is given to staff who come with experience, and flexibility is offered in the selection of workshop experiences.

Associate Degree Graduate Program. Opportunity is available to the graduate of the associate degree program (the staff nurse I) to attend a special development program based on the individual's interest and leadership potential. The twelve-week orientation program provided staff nurse I focuses on basic nursing skills, clinical content, assessment of patient needs, and nursing care planning and evaluation. This orientation is followed by continued centralized and decentralized assistance in beginning leadership skills with approximately 40 hours of formal workshop instruction. Workshop content includes topics such as delegation and accountability, reporting, establishing priorities, the leader and the workgroup, and teaching and learning. When the select staff nurse I is able to meet the role expectations of the staff nurse II category she may be promoted to that position.

Basic Workshops. New diploma (staff nurse II) and baccalaureate (clinical nurse I) graduates are given the opportunity to attend basic workshops. These basic workshops (three 8-hour days) are designed to assist the registered nurse in fulfilling the role expectations held for the teacher and administrator of nursing care (team leader). The primary focus is on providing nursing care through others.

Content in these basic workshops includes sessions on the leader and the work group, observing and recording clinical performance of other staff members, personnel motivation, coping with the authority role of the team leader, developing personal objectives, and teaching and learning. Even though the topics for both workshops are the same, teaching methods used for the two groups are different. For example, we find that the diploma graduates, in general, request more structure to the sessions and supplemental theory related to the topics. Therefore, lectures and discussion reinforced with specifically planned group activities are included in the Staff Nurse II Basic Workshop.

The approach in working with the nurses attending the Clinical Nurse I Basic Workshop is less structured in terms of the theory presented. Problem clinics, which utilize the small group process for problem solving, enable the participants to apply the theory they bring from their educational programs.

Promotional Workshops. Promotional workshops are provided to assist the staff nurse II in fulfilling the role expectations of the clinical nurse I and the clinical nurse I in fulfilling the role expectations of the clinical nurse II (formerly the assistant head nurse position).

Content and general approach to the Staff Nurse II Promotional Workshop is similar to that of the Clinical Nurse I Basic Workshop (three 8-hour days). The additional experience of the staff nurse II in the clinical setting prior to workshop attendance is considered by the instructor when choosing methods of instruction.

Topics in the Clinical Nurse I Promotional Workshop (four 8-hour days) are performance appraisal, motivation, disciplinary approach to personnel problems, guiding and counseling personnel, socioeconomic-cultural factors in the work setting, teaching and learning, and effecting change in the work setting. This content is presented and discussed in greater depth than that in the Clinical Nurse I Basic and Staff Nurse II Promotional Workshops.

Senior Clinical Nurse Workshops. A basic workshop series is offered senior clinical nurses who are relatively new in their roles. These groups tend to be small, allowing for considerable flexibility in planning learning activities. For example, the opportunity was made available for five new senior clinical nurses to develop a videotape production based on changing attitudes of team members about patient care assignments. They wrote the script; role-played the situation; developed objectives, guidelines, and evaluation tools for use of the tape; and shared the tape with their nursing staffs.

Continued workshops are also held quarterly for senior clinical nurses from all clinical services regardless of tenure. Since the major part of their leadership development is provided on a decentralized basis, the programs are often of a general nature. Example topics are: counseling personnel, group intervention, socioeconomic-cultural factors in the work setting, and helping the new registered nurse to assume her leadership responsibilities.

Use of Resource Persons

A wide variety of resource persons participate throughout the leadership development program. Senior clinical nurses, nurse clinicians, directors and assistant directors, faculty from the nursing school, and staff development instructors are involved in the various sessions. Choice of the resource person depends on the specific needs of the learning group, the interest and abilities of the resource person, and the teaching method desired, for example, group problem solving versus lecture and discussion.

One special way in which clinical resource staff participate is through the problem clinics. These sessions are included in the Clinical Nurse I Basic and Staff Nurse II Promotional Workshops and are designed to help the participants to use the problem-solving process in working through their own problems. Two 3-hour sessions are planned, each with a separate focus: the first, to examine the problems in providing quality nursing care to patients; and the second, to analyze difficulties experienced in adjusting to the authority role of the team leader.

The participants are asked to submit a problem related to each of the above-mentioned topics. Problems presented frequently relate to difficulty in holding team members accountable for nursing care delegated, in integrating themselves as the newly hired team "leader" into a stable group of team members, in utilizing effectively the health care resources available to patients and staff, and in collaborating and communicating effectively with the medical staff.

Effective use of the problem-solving approach requires a data base. Therefore, each member is asked to write a description of the character of the clinical unit in which he practices, including information such as census, pace, general acuity level, patient population, predominant leadership style, expectations of followers by leaders and vice versa, and a description of groups and subgroups.

The group is encouraged to be self-directive in helping individual participants work through their problems, especially in identifying alternative solutions. The resource person is available to question, clarify, and answer questions as the need arises. Using resource persons who are involved in the same "real world of nursing" as the participants supports and makes the problem-solving process more realistic.

Considerable effort is expended in creating a climate in the work setting in which individuals have the freedom to question beliefs, policies, and procedures. However, participants in the workshops are continuing to express problems in seeking needed guidance and establishing open and honest communication with their senior clinical nurses. This problem obviously is not unique to nursing as one reviews the literature in an effort to find suggestions for solution.

One important aspect of our workshop program is the opportunity for individuals to have guidance as related to their clinically oriented personal goals. Staff development instructors and senior clinical nurses participate in providing this needed counseling. Participants are expected to pursue their own course of action in solving problems.

The problem clinics are an approach which provides us, as teachers and administrators, with some fascinating evidence of the needs of our registered nurse staff. This information helps us in planning future workshop content. It also has implications for feedback to faculty who are preparing nurse graduates, as well as feedback to senior clinical nurses, directors, and assistant directors, and clinicians who are responsible for planning clinical orientation and continuing education opportunities.

Content Building

Content building from workshop to workshop is one of the major features in a leadership development program when promotional workshops are offered. A particular topic may be included in the Staff Nurse II Basic, the Staff Nurse II Promotional, the Clinical Nurse I Basic, and the Clinical Nurse I Promotional Workshops. Because of differences in role expectations held for the workshop participants as a group, the focus of the content is different for each group. For example, consider the topic of performance appraisal, which is a part of all the workshops listed above.

It is an expectation that staff nurse II and clinical nurses I and II are involved in self-evaluation, including the defining of personal goals related to their clinical responsibilities. Additionally, they are expected to participate with the senior clinical nurse in evaluating clinical performance of other nursing personnel.

The focus in the Staff Nurse II Basic Workshop is examination of the various means of objectively observing and recording the performance of others. Participants submit examples of anecdotal records which are critiqued in terms of factual data collected, interpretations made, and action taken. They discuss the importance of offering immediate feedback to staff members in order to either reinforce or change behavior.

The Staff Nurse II Promotional and Clinical Nurse I Basic Workshop participants are expected to begin working intensively with a select nursing staff member or members on an ongoing basis, and eventually to be involved in helping to compile the formal evaluation. They need to analyze the "system" their own senior clinical nurse has established for carrying out performance appraisal based on information such as when and how are observations of nursing staff shared and with whom? They need also to make plans for working with "their" staff member, to gather data from others, to become more familiar with the categories included in the formal appraisal form, and to set up an efficient record-keeping system for themselves. Discussion and learning activities in these workshops help to prepare the participants in these specific areas.

The clinical nurse II is responsible for actively sharing in the appraisal process with the senior clinical nurse on their unit. In workshop they analyze the system as to flexibility and effectiveness and practice coordinating their anecdotal data into a comprehensive appraisal. Even though formal counseling is considered a part of the appraisal process, it is treated as a separate topic in the Clinical Nurse I Promotional Workshop. Participants have an opportunity to plan and role play a counseling session and then to analyze and evaluate it. Videotaping of the counseling session is sometimes used as a supplemental audiovisual aid.

Teaching methods vary from workshop to workshop along with content focus. Learning activities in the sessions vary from problem solving to triad buzz sessions, small group or individual work, role play, and simulated games. A wide variety of audiovisual aids such as movies, filmstrips, overhead transparencies and audio and videotapes, are available to the learners.

Reference building is an important part of content building, just as varying teaching methods make workshop sessions more interesting and effective. Literature related to each workshop topic is reviewed and considered by staff development instructors. This literature is "graded" for a single workshop group, depending on the focus of the content. This method seems to be more meaningful to the participants than the system of using all available references for all sessions considering a single topic.

DECENTRALIZED REINFORCEMENT OF CENTRALIZED WORKSHOP CONTENT

Many persons are involved in decentralized reinforcement of centralized workshop content, for example, senior clinical nurses, directors and assistant directors, nurse clinicians, and faculty members. Of the various approaches usually taken to this follow-up, one example exemplifies the uniqueness of our organizational structure. One of its basic concepts is that the faculty of the school of nursing will give leadership in the hospital setting by maintaining expertise in their clinical specialty through sustained direct patient care involvement. In turn, the hospital staff has the opportunity to learn from the faculty by utilizing their knowledge and skill in solving patient care problems [3].

The psychiatric nurse faculty, for example, are involved in a series of centralized conferences for senior clinical nurses and clinical nurse II's as resource persons to the individual clinical units. The conferences are aimed at helping these nurses increase their group interactional skills and knowledge of human behavior.

Following theory presentation the faculty lead discussions that help participants examine their own behavior in the work setting. Behavioral concepts such as anxiety, frustration, and hostility are explained in depth. Participants specifically examine their effect on others, describe their own feelings, and identify how they manifest needs through behavioral patterns.

They then move to discuss staff and patient problems related to socioeconomic-cultural factors and how they influence the behavior of the work group. The problem-solving approach is used in an effort to help staff members understand their feelings in a variety of situations. In the centralized workshops they also present concepts of group dynamics and staff counseling. Basic principles of group theory and counseling are demonstrated through role play, audiovisual tapes, and group problem solving.

The psychiatric nursing faculty who participate in the centralized workshops also serve as resource persons to the various clinical units at University Hospitals. Decentralized conferences are held for the purpose of assisting staff to integrate the psychosocial and physical aspects of patient care. Conference discussion concentrates on assessing the psychosocioeconomic-cultural needs of patients and their families, assisting staff to further understand human behavior in relation to the stress of illness.

Another function of the faculty resource person is to assist the senior clinical nurse with her leadership skills in helping staff identify and meet psychosocial needs manifested in patient behaviors. In order to effectively guide the staff toward this end, the senior clinical nurse must have the understanding of individual staff behaviors (including her own) as well as expertise in relating to the group as a whole.

Development of a Planned Conference System

The original plan for conferences was to have the senior clinical nurse contact the psychiatric faculty for psychosocial nursing care problems as needed. Conferences were then scheduled on a prn basis. Individual conferences with the senior clinical nurse to discuss staff problems were also a part of this decentralized plan. In evaluating prn conferences, several negative aspects were found. Frequently, request for conferences came when the patient was ready to be discharged and the plan devised for his care was not used. However, sometimes staff needed to air feelings about the problems rather than utilize help with a specific plan.

With prn conferences, an air of mutual distrust sometimes prevailed, with staff asking help for problems already solved, thus seeking approval for their quality of care. Another disadvantage in having conferences on a prn basis was the lack of opportunity for feedback on nursing interventions and revision of plans. The staff could not always bring appropriate closure to the meetings.

A lack of sufficient data was also a factor in prn conferences. Staff came ill-prepared and were often amazed at the distortion of mutual perception and the amount of conflicting data collected.

As a result of the evaluation of this initial system, the assistant directors, the senior clinical nurses, and the psychiatric faculty decided to schedule weekly conferences with the staff. Currently, conferences are scheduled regularly and specific patients with psychosocial problems are discussed; nursing care is planned accordingly. This idea is readily accepted by the staff. The number of prn calls have been drastically reduced from four or five per week to one or two a month. The senior clinical nurse and staff are able to plan ahead for presentation of patients. Staff members focus on patients' problems and the weekly schedule affords more time to collect data. Regularly scheduled weekly conferences provide a structured opportunity for the staff to share ideas, learn from each other, and evaluate approaches to psychosocial needs of patients. Favorable responses to these scheduled conferences have been received from senior clinical nurses who have the opportunity to utilize a resource person regularly and who now meet with the staff on a planned basis.

Focus of Decentralized Conferences

Using the problem-centered approach, all members of the staff are urged to present patients whom they believe have psychosocial nursing care problems. Initially the senior clinical nurse presented the patients; later, with encouragement, other staff members began to present patients to the group. The senior clinical nurse has the difficult task of guiding staff to collect and share data about patients. It is not unusual for conflicting data about the same patient to be presented in conferences. The need to gather data from all shifts and types of staff in order to complete the picture of a patient and locate the focus of his problems is made quite clear. As the senior clinical nurse leads the conferences, she becomes more adept at helping staff collect and share pertinent patient data and reinforce application of the concepts and dynamics around psychosocial aspects of care.

Some conferences are focused on specific patients while others are not. In the latter, the format is loosely structured and patients are discussed in relation to their total psychosocial adjustment to care. Often these patients are presented in future conferences because the data base has been insufficient for constructing a workable care plan.

It is not unusual for staff problems to emerge during the conferences. These are often worked through while continuing to focus on the patient. At other times, it is necessary to concentrate on the "hidden agenda" of the staff in order to facilitate movement toward devising a plan of care for the patient. Certainly the staff brings with them a variety of socioeconomic-cultural values, beliefs, and opinions that may well interfere with a consistent plan of care for the patient. There are several schools of thought regarding group conferences: (1) Center discussion on patient care and indirectly help staff with their own problems; (2) deal directly with staff problems and then move to patient care problems; and (3) focus intermittently on both staff and patient problems. Just which method is best depends mainly on the leader's philosophy, ease in guiding the conference, and the type of problem manifested. Whether the primary focus is on patient or staff problems does not matter as long as both are resolved—the method of choice rests with the group leader. In our hospital all three approaches are utilized. The following are examples of the three different approaches.

Conference Centered on the Patient's Problems. The following history of a 17-year-old black patient was shared with the faculty integrator during a conference.

> The patient had been readmitted for resuturing of an incision for an appendectomy he had undergone the week before. Apparently he and his brother had been fighting at home and the incision had opened. On this admission he easily irritated the staff by boasting of his endeavors in the ghetto (pushing dope, etc.). He had been shot in the leg during a street fight and walked with a decided limp. The staff assigned him the status of "sinister character." On his previous admission he

had been permitted to visit in the waiting room and had become accustomed to this privilege. The staff did not permit him the same privilege on this admission as they feared he would "get drugs." Because he talked about drugs the staff also became reluctant to give him prn q4h pain medication following surgery and became annoyed when he cried out in pain in less than the 4-hour interval. He also would remove his incision dressing when the pain became intense. The staff questioned whether he was deliberately trying to infect his wound. They also complained about his late night radio playing and voiced concern that he disturbed his white roommate. The staff's solution at this point was to move him into a room with an older black male patient whom they believed would serve as a father figure.

The faculty integrator purposely focused the remainder of the conference on the patient rather than on the staff's attitudes and values. The work group's attitude toward the patient changed as they began to gather more data and assess his needs and strengths. Further collection of data revealed that most of his boasting was about fictitious adventures. He was an innocent victim of a gun battle and in fact had worked very hard to be able to walk again. In spite of physical difficulty, he continued going to school and had plans to graduate from high school. Since his parents were concerned about him, there was little need to provide him with a father substitute. In addition, his white roommate was not disturbed by the radio playing. It was reported that the patient also responded positively to a registered nurse teaching him about contamination of his wound.

The senior clinical nurse used the opportunity to help guide the staff and to examine some of the norms the group held for a 17-year-old boy. They were able to realistically examine his physiological need for pain medication following surgery, along with his reaction to anxiety and their negative responses to him. The staff concluded that he need not be transferred and discussed a plan of care appropriate for his level of development.

Conference Centered on Staff Problems. On another surgical unit, the nurse integrator became involved in a series of planned conferences. The staff was obviously having difficulty communicating with each other and subsequently carrying out planned assignments. The conflict had been going on for some time, but apparently became volatile soon after a young clinical nurse II had been promoted to the senior clinical nurse position. There was a great deal of bickering among the staff and some "acting out" through absenteeism and constant griping. There seemed to be a split between the professional and auxiliary staffs to the extent that the groups strictly adhered to separate coffee break hours.

The first conference was high in interaction as both sides openly expressed feelings and presented their views of the work group's situation. The outcome of the first conference was to establish a series of weekly meetings to help staff analyze their problems. During subsequent meetings, led by the senior clinical nurse with the psychiatric integrator as a

resource person, the group examined personnel policies such as vacations, rotating shifts, seniority, promotions, and holiday time (which seemed to be a very important issue). The group was also concerned about the roles of various staff members and work assignments. After several conferences, the tone of the group began to change, interactions became meaningful, and solutions were based more on reality. Helping the members express themselves in the group was beneficial, communication became open, and decisions were made with health peer group pressure. Staff members seemed more cordial to each other and were enthusiastic about the conferences.

Once the staff was able to work through their own problems, they were ready to discuss patients and patient concerns. They suggested to the senior clinical nurse integrator that the first clinical topic be centered around dying patients. A film on dying was shown and discussed in relation to patients on their division. The senior clinical nurse continued conducting these weekly meetings, using the resource person on a prn basis.

Conference Centered on Both Staff and Patient Problems. The demanding patient is a difficult person to work with, even though specific interventions have been identified for working with this type of patient. Regardless of our knowledge of the dynamics of aggressive behavior, staff seem to need to verbalize their frustrations in caring for each of these patients. In a conference where the demanding patient is presented, the group leader considers the feelings and reactions of staff and realizes that their emotional involvement is unique for each patient. Staff feelings and reactions are considered in developing a plan of nursing care with the recognition that negative attitudes interfere with the transfer of knowledge about one patient to the care of another with similar dynamics.

A. T., a middle-aged female, was in a body cast following back surgery and became very demanding of staff. Her demanding behaviors included ordering detailed care for her flowers and calling her doctor if staff attempted to set any limits. The staff felt frustrated because of the amount of time spent in the patient's room and the patient's use of delaying tactics. The psychosocial, economic, and cultural needs of the patient were discussed in relation to the nursing care problems, as were the concepts and dynamics of anger and hostility related to the staff's feelings in caring for a demanding patient. A plan of care was defined which would saturate her demands and provide a stable care giver who could gradually set limits on her behavior. One registered nurse volunteered to work with the patient during the coming week.

At the following conference the registered nurse said that she was now even more frustrated, although the group was eager to comment on "how much better the patient was." The registered nurse agreed that the patient was less demanding and that she found her to be a really nice person, but at this point, the patient did not want other staff members to care for her. The group was supportive in their comments to the registered nurse, and the senior clinical nurse led the staff in a discussion as to how they might introduce another staff member to the patient in order to alternate care.

Individual Centered Conferences with the Senior Clinical Nurse. The psychiatric nurse integrator also spends time with the senior clinical nurse after conferences reviewing the sequence of events occurring during the meetings and examining group process and progress. Time is also planned periodically for the senior clinical nurse to discuss individual counseling of her staff, anecdotal notes, and other behavioral concepts presented in centralized staff development workshops.

EVALUATION OF CENTRALIZED WORKSHOPS

The process of evaluation is essential to maintaining a vital leadership development program. A formal tool recently has been developed to facilitate feedback from participants and senior clinical nurses regarding change in clinical performance as a result of workshop attendance. In addition, directors, assistant directors, and nurse clinicians share evidence from the clinical setting that workshop attendance has influenced the performance of the participants. Feedback to instructors is shared in formal group discussion, informal individual conferences, and through written materials such as the first performance appraisal prepared by a new senior clinical nurse, anecdotal records compiled by a clinical nurse I, or clinically oriented personal goals written by a clinical nurse II.

Participants in the centralized workshops are asked to appraise the conference (content, teaching methods, useful-ness, etc.) immediately following each session as well as at the end of the total workshop. These responses are used as a guide for program revision. Following each workshop series, the instructor shares information in writing about the participants with their clinical directors. Comments pertain to attendance, a description of the group, participation in discussion and group work, preparation and writing of assignments, and suggestions for the senior clinical nurse regarding planned follow-up.

Occasionally major differences become apparent between what is being discussed in the workshops and what is currently practiced on the clinical units. When this occurs, the instructor becomes involved with the directors, assistant directors, and senior clinical nurses in an attempt to resolve the differences. Decisions are made as to whether the role expectations or the workshop objectives need to be revised.

If workshop participants are not held accountable for utilizing workshop content in the clinical setting, the instructor may need to attend senior clinical nurse meetings or division staff meetings to interpret the problem and to help staff to resolve it. Usually all that is needed is the information that a problem does exist, and the group members respond positively and plan to change the way in which they are holding individuals accountable.

REFERENCES

1. MacPhail, J. *An Experiment in Nursing: Planning, Implementing and Assessing Planned Change.* Cleveland: Case Western Reserve University, Frances Payne Bolton School of Nursing, 1972, p. 61–62.
2. Ibid., pp. 94–95.
3. Pierik, M. M. Experiment to effect change. *Supervisor Nurse* 2(4): 69, 1971.

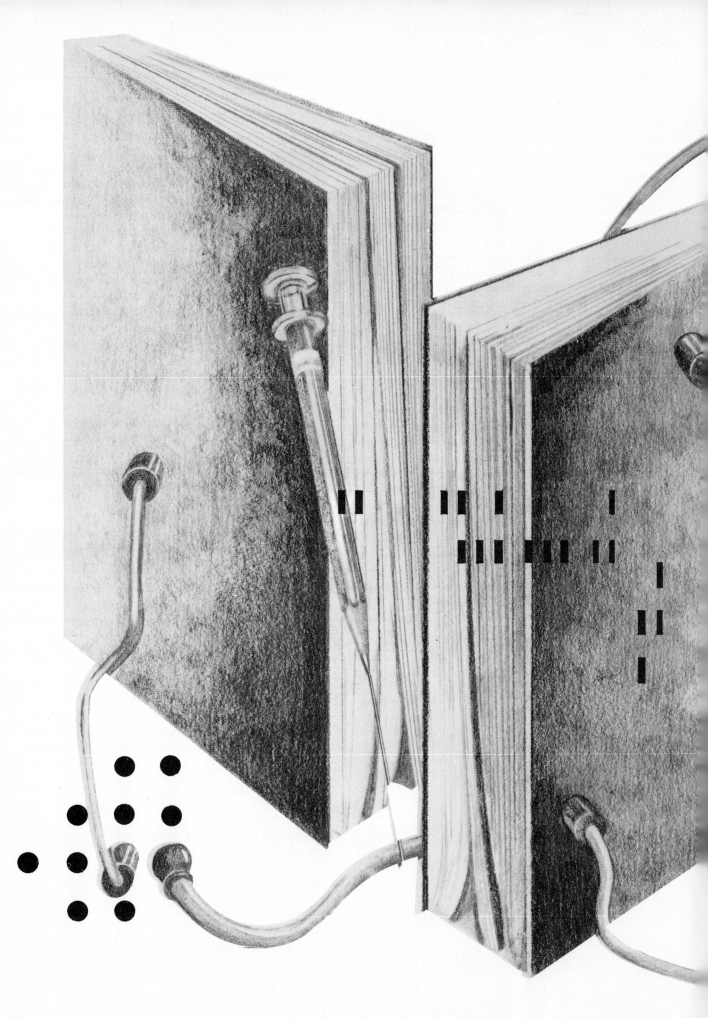

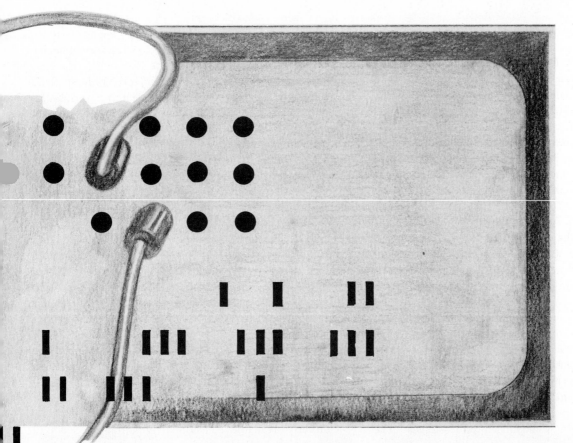

Patricia Hatfield, R.N., M.P.H., is public health nursing consultant, Michigan Department of Public Health, Lansing, Michigan. This article is reprinted from JONA, November-December, 1973.

Continuing education for professionals, particularly for nurses, is recognized as necessary to ongoing viability within the health care system. Imperative questions related to the goal of improved patient care, to the theories of adult education, to the impact on costs to patients, institutions, and practitioners, and to the professional resources available for both service and educational needs are posed. Alternative methods for strengtheneing the performance of nurse practitioners are discussed.

MANDATORY CONTINUING EDUCATION

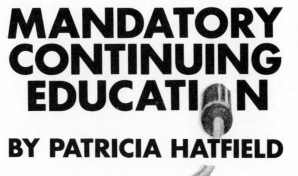

BY PATRICIA HATFIELD

Currently the health profession is one of the services singled out by society for close scrutiny and challenge as to its effectiveness in the health care system. Educators and public school systems appear to have just preceded the health care system in public attention to their inadequacies. Usually these periods of appraisal arise from what is defined as a "crisis" and receive attention from sociologists, legislators, consumers, and dissatisfied members of the profession. The result of all this attention is that problems are identified and categorized, and a multitude of solutions are hastily proposed. Once the identified solutions enter the stage of action, however, little effort is directed toward evaluation, and public concern moves on to other problems within society.

Such terms as *competency-based programs, responsibility, accountability,* and *peer review* reveal the underlying belief that greater effort on the part of the individual practitioner will result in improvements within the system. While this may be only one aspect of the problem, there is a tendency to pin our hopes on the belief that if the proposed solution is generally considered to have merit only good can result. While, undoubtedly, some good may result from a solution idealized as being meritorious, this appears to be a simple approach to a complex set of closely interrelated factors in a system as massive and complex as the health care industry.

The solution currently being promoted within many of the health professions carries the title *continuing education,* or *life-long learning.* Nursing has taken up the challenge and is exploring the promotion of requiring continuing education for licensure. Before we embark on a program for correction of a problem such as the knowledge base of the practitioner, some difficult questions should be explored. Basically, two questions need to be examined in relation to the continuing education issue: (1) Presuming that improved patient care is the objective, would mandatory continuing education credits enable nursing to achieve this goal? and (2) Would requiring continuing education credits ensure that learning takes place, that attitude changes occur, or that new skills are developed?

In attempting to answer these basic questions, four subquestions arise: Is requiring continuing education based on educationally sound principles? What problems are foreseen in relation to implementation of mandatory continuing education requirements? What are the possible consequences of the action? Are alternative methods currently available for meeting the objective?

These questions are not intended to be all inclusive but rather to be a beginning exploration of the topic.

Although the purpose of this article is to oppose mandatory continuing education, this stance should not be interpreted as opposition to continuing education. There does not appear to be any justification for arguing against the need for life-long learning in the professions within society today. Scientific discoveries, technological advances, and increasing knowledge far outstrip our ability to assimilate and act upon new information. There is an ever-widening gap between what is known and what is practiced among the most advanced professionals. The nurse who has not made a real effort to keep pace with new knowledge is hopelessly committed to a traditional but obsolete pattern of nursing care that has not been discarded because systems continue to move in conservative patterns long after knowledge has highlighted the ineffectiveness of current behavior. A professional in any field must engage in activities designed to reduce this knowledge-practice chasm in order to keep his practice relevant and future-oriented.

RELATED EDUCATIONAL PRINCIPLES

Educational theory indicates that adults learn best when objectives appear relevant to their needs. Problem-solving situations provide the opportunity for knowledge to be applied to a specific need of the practitioner, and through this process application is required. When a person tries to apply a theory in the practice setting, new learnings are generated and new insights are gained.

Secondly, intrinsic motivation is more productive than extrinsic motivation. The learner who recognizes and seeks educational opportunities because he visualizes values that meet his needs or because he experiences feelings of competency enters into the educational experience looking for ideas, new modes of operation, or solutions to particular problems. He is an explorer, and the goal of his exploration will be more clearly focused. The individual who seeks educational experiences to satisfy legal requirements may be less actively engaged in the activity. His goal is more tangential to his personal needs, and the resultant attitude may be one of criticism of material presented, less selectivity of the material to be learned, and generally less involvement in the learning process.

Third, new learnings need to be applied. Many continuing education opportunities consist of a series of speakers who inform the audience of the necessary clinical information. The learner is then presented with the task of identifying how this knowledge relates to his practice, how to change practice within his institution, or how to communicate with coworkers in order to implement new learnings.

There needs to be identification of learner needs. Does the learner just need additional knowledge, a change in attitude, or the development of a skill? Each of these activities would require a different educational approach. The learner needs immediate feedback and opportunity for clarification or redirection before he inadvertently applies misinterpreted or partially understood principles. Many educational offerings have been discarded hastily because the learner tried to apply the new knowledge or skill and failed. This can be due to misunderstanding, lack of skill development, only partial recognition of the total process, or even a lack of desire to achieve the outcome [1].

Currently available educational opportunities seem to lack many of the educational principles just described. Primarily, little effort has been made to discover what the learner needs, little opportunity has been provided for practice and feedback, and limited or no support is given the learner as he tries to incorporate new knowledge into practice.

PROBLEMS IN IMPLEMENTATION OF MANDATORY EDUCATION

A decision to require ongoing education for continued licensure has serious implications for nursing practice. Before undertaking a legal course of action, consideration should be directed to the following eight questions related to implementation of a mandatory system of continuing education.

First, how would continuing education be defined? At present there is no universally accepted definition, although there are some proposed ones. California has passed a law which creates a Council of Continuing Education for Health Occupations, and their mission is to establish requirements for continuing education. At this point there does not appear to be a clear definition within the law of what continuing education means,

After January 1, 1975, an applicant for renewal will be required to submit proof to the board that he has informed himself of developments in the R.N. field in the renewal period, either by pursuing an approved course or courses of continuing education or by other means deemed equivalent by the board or by passing an examination [2].

Would college credit be awarded continuing education units or will only noncredit activities be included? The American Dietetic Association has determined that a graduate degree will be counted toward their requirements for continuing education units. Cooper indicates that,

In the broadest interpretation, continuing education encompasses all those learning activities that occur after an individual has completed his basic education . . . Sometimes, however, those educational activities leading to a baccalaureate or advanced degree are excluded from the definition, even though the activities themselves can be seen as part of the individual's continuing education [3].

When currently so many RNs are graduates of diploma schools of nursing, it would seem incompatible with educational goals to withhold continuing education credits for acquisition of a degree. Would professional activities such as attendance at professional meetings, inservice meetings, committees, journal clubs, written papers, talks presented, or personal reading of journals be included? When the above list is reviewed, with the exception of college courses, many problems arise in relation to how standards could be set from which activities could be judged to be acceptable for continuing education units. Many professionals spend a great deal of time reading literature related to their specific needs, adapting these learnings or modifying ideas, and then incorporating them into practice. This type of reading has the advantage of being less time consuming than some other activities might be. If the magazine is in the possession of the reader, four or five articles might be reviewed in an hour. If the learner must journey to a meeting, three or four hours might be consumed. In addition, the meeting may or may not meet the needs of the learner. If the article is not useful the learner has wasted only a fraction of his time.

Would only nursing topics be allowed credit? Many nurses have interest in other fields that would be directly related to their practice but would not be considered nursing topics. Nurses involved with computerized systems of recording or processing data might be very interested in a seminar or lecture on programming a system. A nursing director might be attracted by educational offerings entitled "Management by Objectives" or "Organization Development," and these might be sponsored by organizations within management.

How will we provide for speciality practice? In order to make career goals flexible, would a specialist need to take continuing education credits of a more general nature in order to ensure that she could change areas of practice if she desired? If the nurse in an intensive care unit limits herself to educational offerings most relevant to her current practice, which would strengthen her knowledge in a specialized area, is she circumscribing a limited role for herself?

Fourth, how will the inactive nurse meet the requirements? How will she be informed of continuing education offerings? Would she be able to pay for continuing education when she does not have income of her own? Would she be allowed to let her license lapse and then be relicensed on the basis of an examination? Would this result in a loss of nurses because of their fear of testing after a period of inactive status? Probably the most difficult problem for the inactive nurse would be how to define what will be useful to her in the years to come should she decide to return to practice after a ten- to twenty-year period away from the field.

Will prior approval be necessary for activities of an educational nature, or would subsequent approval be granted? Who would make this determination? How will units be tabulated and who will be responsible for maintaining a record for each individual?

How will the quality of the educational offerings be monitored? Whose responsibility will it be to judge the merit of a program? The most relevant evaluation measure would be change in an individual's practice which results in improved patient care. The means for measuring the benefit to an individual who participates in a workshop or a conference are not available. We can ask her to evaluate her response to the presentation or the unit of study, but change in attitude or acquisition of new knowledge does not necessarily result in changes in performance. There may be a wide gap between what an individual knows and what he is able to do.

Seventh, who will pay for the continuing education? Presently many institutions pay the cost of education for employees, but usually this is on a selective basis and may not involve each individual employed during any one year. Some institutions offer inservice education, and in this way assume the cost. Cost is not always limited to registration fees, luncheons, and travel but must include the cost of released time for employees. If the individual bears the expense, will this mean loss of pay as well as the other expenses incurred? Will the individual who works part-time find that the cost in addition to those of baby-sitting, additional clothing, or the purchase of another car may negate any anticipated income?

Lastly, what standards will be applied in regard to licensing? Will enforcement result in loss of licensure for some individuals? Gearien, in examining mandatory continuing education for pharmacists, states,

We can deny licensure only if the lack of continued education renders the practice of an individual detrimental to the health and welfare of his customers and patients. Thus continued education for maintaining licensure must be based only on the public health responsibility of the pharmacist. To deny a license would put the burden of proof upon the state board and if challenged would have to prove that the pharmacist was incompetent . . . not the pharmacist to prove himself competent [4].

If the nurse does not participate in a workshop or seminar, or read an article during the year, does this mean that her practice is unsafe. If she attends four conferences of poor quality is her practice improved? McGriff presents an argument for mandatory continuing education and proposes that we not delay answers to questions like this. In answer to the statement that mandatory continuing education should wait until measurement of effectiveness has been improved, she replies: "When have tools for measuring the effectiveness of any other educational program been totally successful? But should that mean that we should not move ahead [5]?

The basis of her argument seems to lie in her words "totally successful." It would seem that there are programs that identify competence, particularly in those instances in which the learner applies clinical knowledge in a practice setting. The problem with most continuing education offerings appears to be the lack of a mechanism for evaluating results or possibly that changed practice might not be an objective of the offering.

EXPECTED OUTCOMES

Most problem-solving techniques indicate that the possible consequences of either taking an action or taking no action at all be examined before the plan is completed. Expected outcomes should be reviewed for both good or bad results from the intended action.

The first outcome to be anticipated from mandatory continuing education is increased cost to practitioner, patient, taxpayer, and institution. The increase in cost to the practitioner will arise from assuming responsibility for fees, probably an increased licensing fee, and added time away from current responsibilities. The patient will assume part of the cost through the increased costs to the institution which, in part, are placed on the cost of the health service and are recovered from the client or insurance mechanisms. Taxpayers are involved in the cost when federal grants are used to support educational projects, training, or the funding of schools. Increased institutional costs would arise from greater demands on inservice or reduced working time from all employees participating in educational pursuits during working hours. If the employee feels that as a result of increased education her worth to the institution is greater, there may be requests for increased salary.

The second outcome relates to resources. The first resource to be considered are teachers. Will more nursing instructors be needed? Would presently qualified instructors attempt to meet the need, with the possible result that there is a lessening of quality in all areas. Well-qualified instructors are already in short supply in many universities. Often we do not place a high enough premium on the value of a skilled teacher who balances nursing knowledge and educational methods into a coordinated whole that results in a skilled practitioner. Too often it is presumed

that if an individual knows the content he can communicate that content. If the goal is improved patient care, the quality of the program is very important. Would there be an even greater growth of commercially prepared programs? Although some of these programs appear to be well designed, the cost is often prohibitive.

Would the necessity for continuing education credits result in nurses locating near educational centers where opportunities would be more readily available, thus further reducing the supply of nurses in rural areas?

Would the legislature allocate additional funding to state boards of nursing for the additional staff necessary to approve credits, monitor programs, tabulate units, and enforce compliance?

Would some nurses lose their licenses? They could, by not complying with licensure requirements, thereby allowing their license to lapse.

Would mediocrity result? An already motivated and independent learner may be forced to attend educational offerings in order to obtain credit and thereby have to set aside more creative or innovative pursuits due to time limitations. Some professions with mandatory requirements have discovered that you can lead the learner to the program to register but after that she may go downtown shopping.

Will a false sense of security result? Will there be a tendency to feel that since so many educational offerings are being attended, attendance becomes an evaluative mechanism within itself. We are well aware that tabulating activities and compiling costs can be misleading and may result in not truly evaluating outcomes such as improved practice. Whose responsibility will it be to evaluate growth of an individual? By what means can this be done?

Will the practitioner have a misguided appraisal of his own currency of practice and qualifications for employment? Are we misleading the inactive RN into believing that she can remain current by attending continuing education offerings when in effect she does not have any methods for implementation of new learnings other than through volunteer efforts? We risk the danger of unreal expectations on the part of the practitioner which may exceed the objectives for requiring education.

Will the emphasis on college credits or degrees be reduced? If nursing is ever to obtain professional standing, education must be at college level. What other profession lacks this base? Some may argue that achieving professional status is not desirable for nursing. The advantage of a college education, at this point in time, lies in the emphasis on problem solving rather than on knowledge acquisition for its own sake. With this background the graduate is better able to seek out relevant learning experiences throughout life.

Practitioners may become frustrated with new learnings that cannot be applied in institutional settings. Unless the institution is ready to utilize new methods in patient care or there is a plan for the use of employee ideas, the setting will not be available for change in practice.

ALTERNATIVE METHODS OF IMPROVING PATIENT CARE

In examining a concept such as mandatory continuing education, it is not enough to simply oppose the idea. Obviously the discussion related to continuing education has arisen from the awareness that improvements are needed and therefore some attention should be given to how improvement might be achieved if the proposed approach is not implemented.

First, it seems that in nursing we need to commit ourselves to the position that professional nursing education is obtained in a baccalaureate program. There has been much controversy within nursing about this position. Primarily, this controversy arises from having so many educational methods for obtaining an RN. At present no other program offers to the same degree the potential for developing an individual committed to learning as a lifelong process. A broad academic base provides the learner with an appreciation for the use of the mind that a vocational type of training is unable to do, not due to poor quality but to the limited time within which to prepare a practitioner. We need practitioners who can anticipate changes and who can readily implement changes to accommodate new practices and new discoveries.

Universities should renew and intensify efforts toward assisting the student to develop voluntary patterns of self-initiative. There should be a deemphasis on academic standing by further use of nongraded courses. Many students become involved in the all A's syndrome and lose sight of the value of learning; they devote too much time to "psyching out" the instructor. Their rewards then become the grade rather than increased competency. In lieu of this, more emphasis should be placed on the student by identifying learning needs and independent study techniques and methods designed to give practice in self-assistance. This graduate will then have ample guided instruction in self-pursuit of knowledge.

More effort should be put into resolving the longstanding differences between education and service. Neither can exist without the other, and we must come closer to resolving the problems related to a lack of communication about each others needs. Competition, insecurities, and emphasis upon past poor relationships are detrimental to the full utilization of professionals. A spirit of cooperation needs to be generated between education and service by providing the best qualified practitioner that current knowledge permits and by using this individual to the fullest extent of her abilities.

An individual's qualifications should be evaluated upon employment. Hiring the right individual for the right job ensures that there will be less need for costly orientation or lengthy inservice, and less likelihood of having on staff poorly motivated employees, which results in more frequent turnover of personnel. There must be recognition that RNs do not all have the same interests, and where possible, placement should coincide with the nurse's career goals. This will be more advantageous to the institution, the patient, and the nurse herself. There should be more counseling of individuals out of jobs.

Interviewing of an employee should be related to identifying her philosophy, nursing experience, and knowledge rather than on her willingness to work the assigned hours. Too often, in a tight labor market the tendency is to entice the employee into coming to work regardless of suspected deficiencies. How frequently do we hear, "I know from her references that she had difficulties with employees but I really needed a supervisor." A truly good interview would help the prospective employee and the employer to realize that the type of patient care practiced in the institution will be mutually acceptable to both.

The institution should be dedicated to assisting the individual to develop on the job. If this means additional opportunities, there should be a way of securing help for the individual. The supervisor should have a more active role in identifying the individual who provides the best quality nursing service. Too often the supervisor has identified the individual who arrives late or is too long on the coffee break but is unable to state the quality of her nursing care. The supervisor should be able to identify learner needs and what skills would improve patient care in any unit.

Promotions should be based on careful consideration of the employee's development and demonstrated competencies. Too often longevity is the criteria for promotion. There needs to be a matching of functions to be performed with the individual's ability to perform them in order to assure that organizational objectives will be achieved when added responsibilities are delegated. When administration rewards growth and development, it promotes an unwritten philosophy which indicates to employees how advancement is achieved. This can be a powerful motivational force for employees who desire recognition or status based on their own achievement.

When an institution commits itself to a climate in which employees are expected to be challenged in their abilities and to produce a high level of performance, institutional resources must be allocated to assist the employee. Inservice offerings should be so strengthened that the learner needs are identified and various methods of meeting these needs are offered. This means that the inservice coordinator possesses knowledge of educational theory, methods, and skills which she uses to tailor the situation for the individuals. There needs to be follow-up on learnings, and additional assistance if needed. For some individuals, releasing them from duty for an hour or more to research a problem might be indicated. We are willing to send people to workshops but seldom to provide the opportunity for the development of written materials for staff use or independent study.

Promotion is not always necessary for the motivation of an employee. Job enrichment is currently proposed as a useful method for stimulating employees. Not all nurses desire an administrative position, but they would respond well to additional responsibilities related to a particular interest or ability.

Implied in all these alternative methods for improving patient care is the belief that the practitioner will take up the challenge for her own education when she sees that this has benefit to her as a nurse and to the patients for whom she provides care. When a climate of full use of individuals who demonstrate competency is generated, the less-motivated individual either becomes more interested in self-development or becomes dissatisfied with his situation and through natural attrition may locate employment more compatible with his needs.

Preparing independent learners, resolving conflict between education and service, and improving nursing administration imply that the responsibility for improved patient care is a shared one, whereas mandatory education places the entire responsibility on the practitioner. These methods would involve some additional costs, but it is unlikely that the price tag would be comparable with the cost of instituting mandatory continuing education. Even if the burden of responsibility is placed on the individual,

it is doubtful that the desired result would be obtained in the absence of substantive changes within nursing service.

A paradox within our society is that while there is a growing disrespect for the law, we appear to rely heavily on the authority of the law in an effort to accomplish what we have failed to do by other means. It seems that we opt for the simplest method of doing the job, but, it also may be the least effective in making substantive changes. Using law as a recourse may result in conforming to the letter of the law, but the spirit of this law should be that nurses remain current in the knowledge base needed to perform at the highest possible level; this seems to be the function of education, not law, as Thomas Huxley has described: "Perhaps the most valuable result of all education is the ability to make yourself do the thing you have to do, when it ought to be done, whether you like it or not. This is the first lesson to be learned."

Sir Walter Scott said that, "When a man has not a good reason for doing a thing, he has one good reason for letting it alone." Until thoughtful exploration provides us with more definitive reasons for making continuing education mandatory, there seems to be good reason for delaying.

A rededication to baccalaureate education, restructuring of nursing administration and managerial techniques, and greater efforts to motivate employees to voluntarily seek education and engage in problem solving are seen as methods that might have greater potential for improved patient care. These alternatives distribute the responsibility for goal achievement across the spectrum of the nursing system, not just upon the individual practitioner.

REFERENCES

1. Brown, C. R., and Uhl, H. S. Mandatory continuing education: Sense or nonsense? *J.A.M.A.* 213(10): 1660, 1970.
2. Continuing education required in California for license renewal. *Am. J. Nurs.* 72(2): 198, 1972.
3. Cooper, S. S. This I believe about continuing education. *Nurs. Outlook* 20(9): 579, 1972.
4. Kirk, K. N., and Weinswig, M. Mandatory continuing education for the relicensure of pharmacists. *Am. J. Pharm. Educ.* 36(1): 55, 1972.
5. McGriff, E. P. A case for mandatory continuing education in nursing. *Nurs. Outlook* 20(11): 713, 1972.

Continuing Education,
A Service Agency's Response

by *Frances Marcus Lewis*

Frances Marcus Lewis, B.S.N., M.N., M.A., is a doctoral candidate in sociology of education at Stanford University. She was director of inservice education, El Camino Hospital, Mountain View, California, at the time this article was written. This article is reprinted from JONA, March-April, 1974.

The provision for continuing education concerns nurses on the receiving end, nursing educators, and agency administrators. The author outlines one agency's response to the need and provision for continuing education in nursing. All phases of program planning and implementation are discussed within the context of a teaching-learning philosophy, which depicts the nurse as an active, capable individual with the right to influence and direct her own learning experiences.

Continuing education for nurses is a timely issue. California Law A.B. 449 makes evidence of continuing education mandatory for relicensure for both the registered nurse and the licensed vocational nurse.* Whether mandatory or voluntary, provision of continuing education for nurses needs our attention, and a multifaceted program should be considered by both nurse educators and administrators. In response to this issue, our service agency implemented a plan for continuing education.

The specific program offerings of our agency over a nine-month period, some of the planning that went into these programs, and some of the approaches used to evaluate the programs are the scope of this article. All the programs attempted to meet the NLN guidelines for inservice management and leadership training and continuing education categories and utilized the resources indigenous to our agency [1].

The offerings were based on the belief that a learner has the right to influence program offerings, that advancing the nurse's clinical competence is of utmost importance, and that learning can be predicted, measured, and take place within the context of an eight-hour work day.

---

*California Law A.B. 449 is to take effect January 1, 1977. This paper is an adaptation of presentation made at a district California Nurses' Association Meeting, June 6, 1972.

SPECIFIC PROGRAM OFFERINGS

Over the past nine months our agency has offered seven different series of sessions whose content has direct applicability to the clinical area of practice. A brief overview of these offerings follow.

Advanced Methods of Nurse-Patient Interaction

Helping the patient express his fears, questions, and concerns was the focus of this program. Particular emphasis was placed on an open-ended or deliberative approach to nurse-patient interaction. In this method the nurse consciously avoids putting words into the patient's mouth but rather assists him to elaborate his perception. Emphasis was on the actual *application* of this approach within the context of a helping relationship.

Application of Group Principles

The content in this course was related to principles derived from various group theorists. Emphasis was on the use, or application of, group principles in assessing the strengths and weaknesses of a group as they move, or fail to move, toward goals and on the actions of an effective group member that potentially increase the productivity of the group. Application of these ideas on a nursing unit was explored.

Crisis Intervention Concepts

Concepts derived from crisis theory were explored as the basis for nursing assessment, planning, and intervention. Application of these ideas throughout an acute care setting was emphasized.

Self-Awareness, A Movement Toward Individualizing Nursing Care

Exposing one's strengths, uniqueness, and biases was the main focus of this program. This was then integrated information into the nursing routine. Ways to apply this newly acquired self-knowledge to the clinical area were then explored.

The Process of Nursing Care Planning

The logistics of team care planning was the main emphasis of this session series. It is built on advanced skills in nurse-patient interaction and on a problem-solving model. Particular emphasis was placed on moving from patient assessment to preplanned nursing intervention complementary to, and in addition to, the medical plan of care.

Team Conferences, Facts and Fantasies

Focus was on the common misgivings and misconceptions associated with directing a team conference. For example, nurses are shown that they do not need thirty minutes to build a team nursing care plan, nor do they need to have expert public speaking skills to be effective nursing group leaders.

Death and Dying, The Nurse's Response

Emphasis was on increasing self-awareness and applying facilitative verbal and nonverbal statements when interacting with a dying person and his family. Effective and ineffective coping mechanisms were also discussed.

PROGRAM PLANNING

At this point the reader might be asking, "Where did all the ideas for these programs come from?" "What made you choose one topic over another?" The answers to these and related questions are summarized in our schema for program planning.

The ideas for the program offerings got their start from four areas of consideration: the perceived needs of the nurses at our agency, the needs of the nurses as nursing educators assessed them, current and obvious deficits and strengths identified by the nurses and nursing service administration, and current emphases in the literature and in nursing leadership.

Head nurses from all nursing units were interviewed about their unit strengths, what their hopes for their units were, and what problems they experienced. They were remarkably candid. Where possible, the assistant head nurse and the entire nursing staff were asked the same questions.

After studying the explicit and implicit content of these interviews we estimated what learning needs might be the source of the problems the units were experiencing and what areas could be built upon in an educational experience that would enable the units to capitalize on their strengths.

Throughout the program planning, a significant amount of time was spent in reviewing the literature to determine what nursing leadership across the country was emphasizing, as well as to determine the "meat" of the issues the nurses were suggesting in these interviews.

After anticipating the implicit and explicit content of the interviews and, after reviewing the literature, educational goals for each of the units were formulated. Most signifi-

cantly, program objectives according to Mager were formulated [2]. Bloom's taxonomy of objectives for the cognitive domain also was used [3]. These program objectives were stated in specific behavioral terms and listed in chronological order according to which ones would be attained first and then later built upon. After the objectives were formulated, teaching methodologies and strategies were synthesized to facilitate the achievement of the objectives in reasonable instructor-contact time, given the fact that these staff development sessions would be set up for nurses on their units during a regular eight-hour work day. In most cases what resulted was a series of 7 to 12 one-hour sessions per nursing unit and incorporating two or three behavioral objectives per session.

The session objectives and a brief description of the sessions were then given to the head nurses and assistant head nurses on the units for "clearance," a process analogous to the process involved in "contracting" for objectives [4]. An appointment was made with the head nurses and their assistants to discuss these sessions and the meaning of the objectives, what modifications in objectives or content they wanted, and what their roles would be. Would these head nurses want the nursing instructor to work with them so that they in turn could work with their staff? Would they want the instructor to work with them on some of the sessions? Would they want to assume an exclusive learner role?

After head nurse and assistant head nurse clearance and incorporation of their suggestions for revision, the session went to other members of the target group, the nursing team. In some cases the nursing team was not the target group. In these instances the appropriate group was contacted. Again time was spent in exploring the meaning of the sessions and any revisions the participants wanted.

After the two contracting sessions with the head nurses and other learners, the time and spacing for the sessions was established. Each unit established which time block they could use most effectively. The alternatives may be summarized as follows: (1) one-hour sessions twice a week per unit; one nursing team at a time would have the staff development session while the other team covered the patients' call lights; (2) one-hour sessions twice a week during an extended lunch hour; (3) sixty- to ninety-minute sessions every week from 3:30 to 5:00 P.M.; (4) one- to two-hour sessions every week from 7:00 to 9:00 P.M.; or (5) one- to two-hour sessions rotating through times convenient for all three shifts.

The fourth and fifth alternatives were the only exceptions to programs offered during an eight-hour work day. Attendance at these "after hour" sessions was always high even though the nurses were not remunerated. We believe the attendance remained high because the learners themselves had a say as to the nature of the programs offered.

Once the formats with objectives were determined and the calendar for the sessions was established, the sessions began. The sequence of nine steps in program planning may be summarized as follows: (1) head nurse interview, (2) analysis of the interview, (3) literature review, (4) synthesis of objectives, (5) contract established with head nurse, (6) revision of objectives, (7) contract established with target group of learners, (8) revisions of program, and (9) program implementation.

In addition to the actual contact time we experimented with what we call the *learning task*. The learning task is a structured learning experience *between* program sessions. It guides the learner in behavior and reinforces the learning objectives emphasized in the actual session. It also helps the nurse to integrate the newly learned behavior into her work pattern. For example, one session from the series on Nursing Care Planning dealt with the relationship of an individual nurse's philosophy and goals to what she actually thought and said as she answered a patient's call light. The learning task for that particular session required daily logging of her actual thoughts as she approached a patient's room, what she actually said and did when answering the light, and the patient's response. These notes then became the initial focus for discussion in the next unit session.

Two points should be evident. Our service agency is concerned about inservice education affecting measureable goal-directed behavior change and behavior that increases the clinical competence of our nursing personnel. The achievement of behavioral objectives related to the advanced clinical role of the nurse at the analysis and application levels is the primary concern. What should be evident also is that a large portion of the staff development sessions in the agency is decentralized. That is, emphasis is on a target group of learners. The frequency of auditorium-based in-service is low, except where the program objectives justify such a setting. Rather, nurses are invited into an educational experience in a milieu familiar to them. The informal and formal power of their groups, e.g., their nursing team, is used in the teaching strategies of the session formats to maximize learning opportunities.

EVALUATION

The evaluation component of the inservice program is really not the last portion of inservice programs at the agency. Rather, the utilization of Mager's concept of behavioral objectives immediately implies *concurrent* measurement of growth in the learners [2]. The way the objectives are stated gives the instructor an immediate indication during the program session whether the nurses are getting what they need. In this way the instructor does not find at the end of the series that she has "lost" the learners. Also, the objectives are stated in ways that the nurse herself knows what she needs to learn. Thus behavioral objectives become both the beginning and the end of the teaching-learning process. In addition, we have experimented with other forms of evaluation, nonparticipant observation, peer evaluation, participant observation, and self-report.

Our experimentation with nonparticipant observation involved one of the head nurses and her assistant head nurse. An observation tool was specifically designed for their unit and was directly related to the behavioral objectives of their staff development formats. The tool specified nursing behavior with patients and among staff members to be accepted as evidence of achievement of program objectives. We "trained" these two nurses in the use of this tool. The observation periods in which the tool was used were established as before and after the staff development sessions, i.e., timed similarly to a pre- and post-test. The results were mixed because the format of the tool was too abstract for the observers, despite several revisions.

Our findings in peer evaluation have been promising. We have been able to obtain objective evidence of behavioral change by anonymous nursing personnel peer rating by means of an open-ended questionnaire. This was an exciting find because we had thought that peer rating would offer only general evaluative comments.

Evaluation by participant observer has given us some additional information. One head nurse was trained as a participant observer to evaluate her staff's response to their unit's staff development program. She was so eager to have her staff succeed that she had difficulty in maintaining objectivity and specificity as participant observer.

The type of evaluation saved until last is the one we probably all tend to rely on most, the self-report, i.e., what the learner says about himself and what he has learned. In all instances our self-reports gave us evidence of specific and even somewhat detailed behavioral change. We seldom received general responses such as "I learned a lot." Rather, we received statements such as, "I am now better able to help the patient express his feelings about death without getting tense or changing the subject."

In addition to conventional inservice offerings, we have implemented a decentralized approach to inservice—in most cases unit-based programs designed to build upon existing strengths and to work toward problem solutions. In all cases the learners have had an active say in the objectives, content, format, and timing of the sessions. Various types of program evaluation have been tried. We believe that the programs offered and those in progress satisfy stringent criteria for continuing education for relicensure. The programs all speak to the issue of professional growth and competence.

REFERENCES

1. Miller, M. *Inservice Education for Hospital Nursing Personnel.* New York: National League for Nursing, 1958.
2. Mager, R. F. *Preparing Instructional Objectives.* Palo Alto, Calif.: Fearon, 1962.
3. Bloom, B. S. (Ed.). *Taxonomy of Educational Objectives. Handbook I: Cognitive Domain.* New York: McKay, 1956.
4. Blair, K. It's the Patient's Problem—and Decision. *Nurs. Outlook* 19(9): 587, 1971.

Mandatory Continuing Education for Professional Nurse Relicensure. What Are the Issues?

by Barbara J. Stevens

Barbara J. Stevens, R.N., M.A., is an assistant professor of nursing service administration, University of Illinois and a doctoral student, University of Chicago. This article is reprinted from JONA, September-October, 1973.

Mrs. Stevens identifies issues that should be addressed by groups considering the mandating of continuing education for professional nurse relicensure. She examines the objectives offered for legislating continuing education, discusses the problems anticipated in implementing licensure laws, and stresses the need for careful consideration of all aspects before decision-making on the issue.

In virtually every state in our country, professional, commercial, and consumer groups are encouraging the adoption of mandatory continuing education for professional nurse relicensure. California already has passed a law to that effect; several other states have similar bills under consideration. In principle, everyone agrees that continuing education is an essential for the practicing nurse. From this consensus, it is easy to move to the concept of mandatory continuing education in order to assure that each nurse fulfills this professional obligation. The move to legislate what everyone agrees upon in principle seems to be a simple and logical progression, but such a transition ought not be considered without addressing all the issues involved.

The author's position in this paper is neither for nor against mandatory continuing education. However, the author is against any such mandate which has not fully considered the issues involved. This paper attempts to identify some of the major issues and problems that should be addressed by any group considering the question of legislating continuing education for nurses.

The first consideration in relation to mandatory continuing education is the purpose behind the trend. Given that continuing education is necessary for the nurse, what is the objective in making it mandatory? If a group has no clear objective in mind, then there is no use in proceeding. If, however, a clear objective can be identified, then one must ask: Is mandatory continuing education the most appropriate way to attain that objective?

MANDATORY CONTINUING EDUCATION TO FOSTER PROFESSIONAL PRACTICE

One common objective given for mandatory continuing education is that of assuring professional practice. One characteristic of a profession is that the practitioners are indoctrinated into a role model that includes self-responsibility for learning relevant to the tasks assumed in professional practice. The fact that nursing groups are moved to consider legislating continuing education indicates an awareness that not all practitioners of nursing are practicing at a professional level. Somehow, nursing has failed to instill an appropriate role model in some occupational members.

The question is not whether this condition exists; it is a fact that many nurses do not maintain professional practice. The important question should be: Is mandatory continuing education the way to solve this problem? Will forced attendance at educational programs change the mind-set of the nurse who has not internalized the professional role model? Will required attendance at educational programs assure that the nurse with this psychology will absorb and transfer new learning to her work situation?

Obviously the solution does not fit the problem. The problem with this sort of nurse is not the lack of specific education per se but lack of an appropriate attitude toward educational obligations. Aiming to "force feed" the nurse does nothing to cure the inappropriate attitude and role model failure. A better approach to the problem would be to develop a system of peer censure and to develop mechanisms whereby nursing departments refuse to retain unprofessional nurses. Continuing education programs aimed at teaching specific nursing content will not resolve the problem of the nurse who does not accept the professional role.

The attempt to mandate continuing education for this objective indicates a failure on the part of nursing as a profession. It is an admission that nursing has been unable to establish control over its own constituent. The move to mandate continuing education is a move to relinquish internal, professional control in favor of external, societal control. There is presently great effort toward the establishment of this external control. One wonders what would have happened if nursing, as a united profession, had elected to put equal energies into the establishment of internal controls instead. This is not to overlook the efforts of some states to establish internal controls at this time, but these efforts are not united and consistent.

MANDATORY CONTINUING EDUCATION TO PROVIDE LEARNING OPPORTUNITIES

Another purpose often cited in support of continuing education legislation is the provision of needed learning opportunities for nurses. Supporters of this position claim that only legal requirements will force employers to make adequate time and money investments in staff education. Legal requirements, also, it is claimed, will provide a basis for investment in continuing education by colleges, universities, health and professional agencies, and commercial organizations.

If provision of learning opportunities is seen as the primary objective of mandating continuing education, several subissues must be considered. These issues involve conceptual as well as operational problems. The first and most important question is the content of the learning opportunities to be provided. Learning opportunities to what end?

The Content Question

There are several possible answers to the content question:

1. The learning opportunity can be any sort of experience that renews and revitalizes the nurse's interest in her profession and in her practice. Its purpose is to stimulate personal and professional growth.

2. The learning opportunity should update the nurse. It should bring her in contact with the newest advances in the field of nursing.

3. The learning opportunity should be such that it helps the nurse improve her actual job performance. It should relate directly to her actual role performance.

The first position is easily recognized as another form of the first objective discussed in this paper, that of mandatory continuing education as necessary to assure professional practice. Role inculcation underlies this viewpoint and is evident in the variety of forms of continuing education which are accepted as valid under this position. If one examines the proposals being drafted by various nursing organizations and groups, this position is usually the one being adopted. Minor differences can be seen from one plan to another; some plans accept formal academic study, some do not. Some accept proof of independent professional activity, some do not. Some give credit for learning which takes place as part of the job, some do not. What unites all these plans conceptually is the credit given for multiple types of learning experiences without requiring that the learning experiences be related to a particular content standard. These plans usually discuss quality of the learning experience, but content is not submitted to stringent criteria. To require that content be nursing-related or even to require that it be some form of nursing itself is not a stringent criterion.

To illustrate how a typical plan of this type functions, nurse X might meet her continuing education requirement by the following happenchance collection of learning experiences: (1) seminar on the dying patient, (2) workshop on how to do nursing care plans, (3) course on care of the geriatric patient, and (4) presenting a paper at an AORN convention. Assuming that these activities added up to the appropriate number of points, the nurse would have her continuing education requirement. The fact that she might be an operating room nurse, who will only minimally use the content of three out of four of the learning experiences, is not considered.

Thus the intent of plans of this kind cannot be related to nursing content or nursing process; the intent must be seen as related to nursing role inculcation. The objective is to keep the nurse inspired, interested, and generally maintaining a professional approach to her nursing career. Arguments have already been offered in the first section of this paper against the suitability of mandatory continuing education for solving problems of role inculcation.

The second position, which bases mandatory continuing education on the need to keep abreast of new developments in the field of nursing, also has some problems. Since this objective is content oriented, it assumes that new, universal content should be given to all nurses. The problem here is operational. Who will decide what nursing content is to have this status? Will it be limited to "hands-on'' nursing care? Can it include trends and nursing systems? Will it include only new aspects that are generalizable to all nursing practice? Or will it include new nursing content relative to special fields of practice? Who will set the criteria by which the essential new nursing content will be selected? The growing specialization in nursing makes it especially difficult to isolate "new" nursing content every nurse should know to be considered updated.

The third position tries to solve this dilemma by relating the content to the individual nurse's job. In order for this criteria to function, it is necessary that each nurse receive continuing education relevant to her particular functional role. The extensiveness of such an undertaking will be evident if one thinks of the multiple functional roles that nurses fill in any one institution. This task would be further compounded by the many different institutional settings in which nurses work. The problem of multiple roles (each role needing its own continuing education) would be further compounded by geographic considerations. Not all nurses would have geographic proximity to others needing education in the same role function. Thus the first problem with matching education to job performance would be the multiplicity of programs needed to even begin to do the job.

A second problem with job-related education would be content selection. For example, content in management techniques might be more relevant for a director of nursing than would be nursing content per se. A nurse in a Spanish-American community might find that studying the Spanish language was the best continuing education for her. What criteria would be established, and by whom, for deciding what continuing education properly relates to job performance and meets the nursing licensure requirement?

Another problem arises when the nurse wants to accept a new role, assuming that continuing education is related to role performance. In switching from pediatrics to adult medicine, for example, would the nurse be limited by her previous continuing education content?

The concept of job-related continuing education has one merit that should be noted: it is easier to justify the financial and time outlay when such education is directly related to improved services for clients.

To summarize the content issue, at least three positions have been identified: (1) education relevant to role inculcation, (2) education relevant to nursing content per se, and (3) education relevant to nursing function. Clearly, other positions could be identified on the role-content-process continuum. For example, one might claim that continuing education aims to give each nurse broader scope of knowledge without relating that increased breadth to job performance or to updating. Such a position is very difficult to justify as a legal mandate, however, since it doesn't identify a necessity for either the nurse or the client. Content,

however, is only one of the issues if mandatory continuing education aims to provide learning opportunities. One must next ask if legislating continuing education will in fact meet the objective of providing more learning opportunities for nurses.

The Provision Question

In every law drafted to date, the ultimate onus is on the nurse herself to find the necessary learning opportunities to renew her license. No law, to the knowledge of this author, has been suggested which requires any agency or organization to provide such experiences. The effects of demand, however, are predictable. Already in the larger cities one sees universities, colleges, professional organizations, and inservice departments making strides in providing more and higher quality programs in continuing education.

The problem in provision is one of equal opportunity. Obviously, areas without universities, colleges, or large professional organizations will have fewer systems available to provide the voluntary increase in continuing education programs. The nurse in the rural setting will have the same licensure demands as the nurse in the city, but she will have fewer resources with which to meet those requirements. Groups seriously considering mandatory continuing education should have a solution to this problem built into the proposed law. Without some provision for equal opportunity, a mandatory continuing education act may cause a shift in the geographic population of nurses. Nurses might show a greater drift toward urban settings so as to be near continuing education centers.

MANDATORY CONTINUING EDUCATION TO PROTECT THE CONSUMER

A third alternative objective offered in support of mandatory continuing education is the need to protect the consumer of nursing services. This same objective is sometimes stated in more positive terms such as "to benefit the client." Again, this is a worthy objective, but one must ask if continuing education can meet this objective, and, if so, under what conditions?

Content related problems have already been discussed, and this objective clearly requires the relation of content to client services. The objective presents another problem which has not been discussed. For the objective of providing learning opportunities for nurses, it was enough that a system brought nurse and program together; for a consumer-related objective, this is not enough. Mere "body-present" at a learning experience is no guarantee that the nurse will absorb new knowledge, let alone that she will apply it in the nurse-client situation. The only way one can judge whether a continuing education experience really benefits and protects the client is to evolve a testing system. Nurses could be tested for knowledge attainment at the end of each learning experience, but this alone would still not identify the nurse behavior in the nurse-client situation. Thus, for meaningful evaluation of learning, the nurse would have to be assessed in her use of the new learning in her actual work situation with clients. Systems would have to be evolved to measure whether the nurse "passed" or "failed" in relation to each learning experience before the experience could go toward meeting her continuing education requirement.

Many continuing education programs are now carrying out such evaluations, but, in general, nursing is not operating at this level of sophistication. The economic impact of extensive evaluation also needs to be considered. Costs would spiral if every workshop or program included assessment of each participant's application of content in her own work setting. To this author's knowledge, no proposed law for mandatory continuing education requires an evaluative process. Therefore no present law can be said to deliver on a consumer-related objective.

OTHER ISSUES

Whatever the objective in legislating continuing education for nurses, certain operational questions must be addressed. Reciprocity in continuing education experiences for the mobile nurse would become a question. Already we have seen different states draft and consider different legislation concerning continuing education. Some proposed laws put continuing education certification under the state board of nurse examiners; some put it under the state nurses association. Others may yet come up with different accrediting bodies. In addition, most systems being drafted do not coincide in their requirements in either content. quality, or amount of work. It would be frustrating to see nurses inhibited in geographic relocation by continuing education requirements as they once were by different state board requirements for licensure. It was a long struggle to get a country-wide examination system; is nursing to begin a similar struggle again?

Reentry problems could also be created by an ill-prepared mandatory continuing education law. What consideration will be given, for example, to the nurse returning to practice after taking time out for family responsibilities or even for further academic education? Would restrictive laws lose some of this population to other fields? Is that loss to be considered productive or counter-productive?

Recruitment into nursing could also be altered by the continuing education mandate. Would nursing lose potentially valuable people to fields with more permanent security, or would the mandate serve to "weed out" undesirables? For the 18- to 19-year-old population considering nursing, can one realistically expect them to react with maturity to the implications of commitment to life-time study?

Self-study is another area that must be considered. Is the system designed to credit self-study? It is likely that self-study is still the dominant mode of continuing education among nurses. How can self-study be measured and credited in a mandated situation?

These questions are but a few with which any group seriously considering mandatory continuing education must grapple. It is not enough to determine that continuing education is a "good thing." Any responsible group must anticipate the conceptual and operational problems likely to occur if that good thing is mandated. It is on the basis of the answers to these problems, rather than on good intentions, that decisions to mandate or not to mandate should be made.

The Continuing Education Unit:
A New Concept of Measurement

by Maryanne E. Roehm

Maryanne E. Roehm, R.N., Ed.D., is professor and director, continuing education in nursing, at Indiana State University, Terre Haute, Indiana. She is a member of the coordinating committee of the Indiana Statewide Planning Committee for Continuing Education in Nursing. This article is reprinted from JONA, March-April, 1974.

The development of a new concept of measurement for continuing education is reviewed. The purpose of the continuing education unit is discussed in light of quality continuing education as a means of improving the nurse's practice.

Society has come to believe that lifelong learning is a right of the individual and an obligation of the professional practitioner. Concomitantly, the necessity for every practicing nurse to update and expand her professional knowledge and skills throughout her career is unquestioned and essential. Nursing also shares with other professions and society-at-large some of the reasons that make it necessary to inaugurate a universal system of measurement for recording participation in nontraditional educational activities that do not lead to a degree. This article discusses the development and purposes of a new concept, the continuing education unit (CEU), as it affects nurses and nursing practice.

WHAT IS A CONTINUING EDUCATION UNIT?

The continuing education unit is a standard of measurement for noncredit education by adults. As defined by a national task force, one CEU equals 10 clock hours of participation in an organized learning activity under responsible sponsorship, capable direction, and qualified instruction [1]. Criteria for continuing nursing education and the assigning of CEUs are being established by the ANA Council on Continuing Education so that the nurse learner can be assured that the CEUs she receives meet national standards.

Thousands of nurses are among the more than twenty-five million Americans participating in informal education each year. Educational institutions currently offering non-credit courses use a system of measurement deemed suitable for their own purposes, thereby causing confusion within the total continuing education effort. With the increasing national emphasis on education throughout a career, the need for a uniform, nationally accepted unit has become

urgent. An official record for this type of learning is usually not available to the learner, as is true of college credit, and there are no reliable data on the quantity or quality of continuing education activities taking place today, since official records are seldom available. As universities become increasingly involved in continuing education, an attempt is being made to systematize programming and credentialing before too many varieties of units are developed and change to a national standard becomes too difficult.

The idea of a uniform, national measurement evoked such great interest that the National Planning Conference of the National University Extension Association, the American Association of Collegiate Registrars and Admission Officers, the U.S. Civil Service Commission, and the U.S. Office of Education created a National Task Force in 1968 to study the feasibility and implementation of a uniform measurement for noncredit continuing education programs. The task force has published statements on the CEU and its administration. Progress reports from pilot projects indicate that the CEU is workable and has the potential of becoming widely used.

Some of the reasons that led the task force to recommend the CEU were that the CEU is decimally related to the instructional hour, which is the most common module of education, that it parallels precedents of the familiar concept of credit, and that it is appropriate for postsecondary through postdoctoral participants. The CEU is easily computed for all courses regardless of format, sponsorship, and duration, and it is applicable to current programs.

Even though the American Nurses' Association is not a member of the task force, the ANA Board adopted the recommendation to use the CEU as defined in the interim statement of the task force. By endorsing the concept, the ANA is committed to the assessment of the unit's potential value for nurses and nursing. Audrey Spector, former Coordinator, Continuing Education, ANA, at the 1971 National Conference on Continuing Education in Nursing, asserted, "the national professional association is concerned with finding the best method of promoting continuing education in a way that will be in the best interests of nurses and of the public" [2].

As further evidence of its commitment, the ANA has approved the establishment of a Council on Continuing Education under the auspices of the Commission on Nursing Education. The Council is designed to carry out the professional association's responsibilities in continuing education. Responsibilities of the Association include encouraging nurses to keep their knowledge and skills current, promoting and conducting scientific sessions, promoting the establishing of programs within the educational system and legislation and funding for programs, and planning with other organizations and associations for coordination of continuing education efforts [3].

Reports of the 1972 ANA biennial convention and statements published during the past year describe a myriad of continuing education activities, reflecting the profession's concern that nurses increase their ability in practice. During the convention an amendment seeking ANA support for requiring evidence of continuing education for relicensure was proposed. This amendment, however, was defeated by the House of Delegates. From a draft of standards for continuing education in nursing shared with members of the convention, an *Interim Statement on Continuing Education in Nursing* has been circulated to members of the ANA Council on Continuing Education, state nurses' associations, state boards of nursing, committees on continuing education, and institutions of higher learning for their review and consideration [4]. The Interim Statement defines continuing education in nursing as systematic learning experiences designed to enlarge the knowledge and skills of nurses. These learning experiences do not refer to education toward an academic degree or preparation of a beginning professional practitioner. "Continuing professional education activities provide more specific content applicable to the individual's immediate goals; are generally of shorter duration; are sponsored by colleges, universities, health agencies and professional organizations; and may be conducted in a variety of settings" [5]. The document lists guidelines for conducting continuing education in nursing and includes a statement on the use of the CEU. From recent information secured on a national survey of continuing education programs available to registered nurses, the ANA can define its role in continuing education. The report furnishes a foundation for planning and further study. Nineteen recommendations in the report cover a wide range of issues [6].

WHAT ARE THE PURPOSES OF CEU?

The CEU was designed as a uniform, nationwide measure for recording and reporting about continuing education. Its use permits the accumulation, updating, and transfer of the individual's record to another individual, to employers, organizations, agencies, and others who require such evidence of continuing education. The CEU is intended to encourage long-range educational goals and continuing education as a process of lifelong learning, make the pursuit of knowledge more attractive as a way of personal and professional development, provide a framework within which an individual can develop at his desired pace, and permit and encourage the adult student to marshall and utilize a host of continuing education resources to serve his particular needs [7].

Possible applications of the unit are short courses, inservice programs that improve competence, and other programs designed to upgrade performance, e.g., symposia, conferences, seminars, institutes, workshops, clinical sessions, and organized independent study. All continuing education offerings do not meet the criteria for assigning CEUs, regardless of their usefulness to the learner. Examples of activities not awarding CEUs might include casual lecture series requiring only attendance, series of disconnected presentations such as topical conferences, general reading, discussion groups, films, attendance at business meetings, committee membership, job orientation, travel, community activities, and courses carrying academic credit. CEUs are not applicable toward meeting the requirements of a degree.

With the prospect of a system of measuring and recording, nurse participants will be encouraged to choose courses that best fit their needs and career goals. They determine the usefulness of each course and choose from among a variety of sponsors the format of the offerings best for their self-improvement. Nurse learners relate CEUs to career goals, and CEUs provide evidence that nurse practitioners accept the obligation to continue to learn. CEUs are evidence to the nurse's clients that she feels a sense of obligation to keep professional service at the highest possible level of performance; CEUs are evidence to the professional association that the nurse accepts the obligation to continue to learn and could be used in states that require evidence of continuing education for license renewal. Courses meeting national standards should be readily acceptable in all states, facilitating interstate mobility of nurses.

The CEU is not to be confused with certification. Recognition of excellence in clinical nursing practice is being achieved through ANA's program of certification of practitioners. Continuing education would be one avenue by which the nurse maintains professional effectiveness, and the record of CEU would be submitted to certification boards for each division of nursing practice to support the claim of excellence in practice. Certification could provide the stimulus for the nurse to enroll in a systematic and orderly set of learning experiences that assist in reaching professional career goals. The ANA has suggested that state nurses' association not engage in certification programs.

State nurses' associations are, however, setting criteria for recognition of continuing education, and evidence of CEUs may be one requirement. In its *Statement of Interpretation and Clarification in the Use of CEU*, the Interim Executive Committee of the ANA Council on Continuing Education for Nursing recently suggested that a point system be devised for various activities each association desires its members to meet, but that the CEU be used only for measuring and recording organized learning experiences [8]. The statement further explains that CEUs might be converted to points for such recognition programs, but that points for activities other than organized learning experiences should not be assigned CEUs. There are state nurses' associations that require continuing education for membership in the association.

Employers need to measure the impact of continuing nursing education activities on the improvement and changes within the health care system. Administrators of nursing services have a special obligation to see that nursing practice is improved. Their greatest challenge is the ability to foster the development of the nurse's capacity for self-development and to remove obstacles that hinder this growth in the work situation. It is the nurse administrator's responsibility to see that the organization is designed to be conducive to the individual nurse's fulfillment. Nurses administering continuing education programs and nurses administering health services must work together to set up objectives that the nurse learner is more apt to apply upon completion of the course.

For the sponsor and nurse responsible for producing continuing education programs, the CEU is a tool for reporting individual achievement and it appears to have the following advantages: (1) it can be applied to any educational experience not applicable toward a degree, (2) it can be used in all learning experiences without regard to format, content, level of audience served, or length of the offering, (3) it can be applied with ease to existing programs, (4) it appears to have respectability and status with academia, and (5) it provides for the collection of statistical data for budget, program planning, and comparative studies within the institution and on a national basis.

HOW IS THE QUALITY OF CEUs CONTROLLED?

Quality control for the assigning and awarding of CEUs is an extremely important matter. Viewed as a system of measurement and recording delineates the CEU in a narrow sense. It discusses the meaning of the concept in quantitative aspects. We need to give attention to the qualitative aspects of continuing education so that nurses can make judgments as to the kinds of CEUs that are desirable.

The key to quality CEUs lies within the definition of CEU—participation in an organized learning experience, under responsible sponsorship, capable direction, and qualified instruction. The *Interim Statement on Continuing Education for Nursing* proposes guidelines for conducting educational programs and for determining whether an offering is worthy of being assigned CEUs. In order to make these standards workable for committees who might be approving courses for the awarding of CEUs, assessment factors for each of the guidelines is helpful. Indiana, through its Statewide Planning Committee for Continuing Education in Nursing, has begun to establish assessment factors for each of its standards. Because Indiana's plan for continuing education is based upon voluntary participation,

Regional Committees of the Statewide Planning Committee have the responsibility for reviewing and approving courses for CEUs awarded in that region.

Organized learning experiences include all institutional learning in organized formats. Learning experiences assigned CEUs must be planned and organized around clearly defined objectives, content and learning activities must be designed to meet these objectives, outcomes must be determined through evaluation techniques, instructors must be qualified, and the learning experiences must be based on the educational needs of the learner [9].

A great degree of latitude is allowed in sponsorship of programs and includes sponsors outside academia. A legitimate sponsor is one who has the authority to offer educational programs. The nurse would not be expected to obtain all courses at any one institution, and no one institution can purvey all continuing education imposed upon the learner. The nurse would be encouraged to use a number of resources to meet well-formulated career objectives.

The sponsor is responsible for establishing and maintaining a permanent record of all CEUs awarded, and individual records are to be available in response to requests. Abstracts of essential information on each course conducted should be filed for satisfying inquiries.

The role of the nurse educator in continuing education is to set up for nurse learners conditions that are conducive to growth and development. It is the primary responsibility of this educator to build quality programs on the existing knowledge and experience of nurse learners and to translate these educational needs into systematic learning experiences. Continuous guidance by a responsible person results in higher quality programs. The nurse educator in continuing education assists the learner to diagnose her needs, includes her in planning course objectives and learning experiences, sets a climate conducive to learning, provides the necessary resources, and assists the nurse learner in self-evaluation [10]. Continuing education clientele need to be kept informed of continuing education opportunities.

Even though the focus of continuing education for nurses is on new knowledge and skills to update practice, quality courses will assist the learner in the application of that knowledge in the work situation. Courses that lend themselves to direct clinical application ought to have planning input from practitioners in those areas. It is a challenge to the nurse educator to meet the needs of nurses and the health care needs of the community.

The teaching staff should be knowledgeable about concepts of adult learning and possess expertise in the content to be presented. Continuing professional education is grounded in a philosophy of higher adult education which, first and foremost, implies one of responsibility of the individual nurse. The profession strives to better itself through the use of active principles of learning to achieve the basic aims of the group [11]. The educational process would emphasize the individual learner in terms of the quality of his experience in an environment in which he finds his own way toward full development. Adult education helps learners to learn for themselves, helps individuals to acquire the skills of self-directed inquiry, and facilitates the accomplishment of desired goals. The test of the value of continuing education is its effect in furthering continued growth and the extent to which every nurse develops into full stature. Continuing education can meet the criterion of education as growing when, and only when, development is conducive to continuous growth of the individual throughout life.

Adult learners are self-directing persons, and their experiences are one of the greatest resources for learning. Social roles of adults have provided them the readiness to learn, and they enter a learning activity in a problem-centered frame of mind. The curriculum is related to solving problems of everyday life and work of the participant. It begins with interest in these problems, and the means through which they are solved requires the active involvement of the learner. Only then is learning meaningful, and only then can the learner experience the rewards of greater knowledge, skills, and understanding.

The only legitimate basis for evaluating a program is its own objectives. All persons who could make a judgment about a particular program should be included in the evaluation process. In addition to the nurse participant, this would include nurse experts in the area and supervisors and managerial personnel who have responsibility for nursing practice in a health care setting. It is appropriate that consumers of health care be involved in planning and evaluating certain programs, and nurse educator in continuing education should include these persons in the planning of course objectives and learning experiences. The continuing educator's collection of data should be pertinent to the nurse's application of learning on the job, including data that might indicate sources of difficulty within the work situation that might hinder job effectiveness. Such data might indicate the need for administrative personnel within the institution to seek assistance with promoting a better work environment.

Because the purpose of evaluation is to stimulate the growth and improvement of the learner rather than for grading purposes, self-evaluation is the most important facet of the evaluation process.

HOW DOES THIS NEW SYSTEM WORK?

Since the administrative process provides the quality control for the units, requirements have been set by the National Task Force for administering the CEU. Procedures will vary with each institution; therefore, only the general process will be discussed. The instructor responsible for each course, in cooperation with the nurse producer of the continuing education program, establishes the appropriate number of CEUs to be attached to a particular offering. Faculty members are more intimately aware of the scope, format, and content of the offering, and the program director is more knowledgeable about the administrative requirements for the course. The number of CEUs awarded to the potential nurse participants would be determined in advance of the offering and would appear on the announcement prior to nurses enrolling in the course.

Continuing education in Indiana is on a voluntary basis. Each regional committee of the Statewide Plan for Continuing Education therefore, will review the course proposals within its region, using the assessment standards developed by the Statewide Planning Committee. It is the belief of the Committee that approval is essential for quality CEUs in nursing. This practice does not deny the use of CEU to anyone, but it does alert the nurse learner that the course has met criteria set up by a recognized group.

The instructor reports to the nurse educator in continuing education the participants who completed each course. The number of CEUs earned by each individual is then certified for the permanent record. A copy of the CEU record may also be provided to the participant and to the employer. The system of CEU records may be related to the current system of permanent records in use at the institution, however. The task force has made suggestions as to the information desired on a record. As a service to its continuing education clientele, the sponsor provides a transcript of the CEU record to any appropriate inquirer. In a recent survey of current continuing education programs, it was recommended that the ANA explore the possibility of developing a national system of recordkeeping using the CEU [12]. It is conceivable that a central national data bank will record all CEUs awarded.

REFERENCES

1. *The Continuing Education Unit: An Interim Statement of the National Task Force.* Washington, D.C.: National University Extension Association, 1970, pamphlet.
2. Spector, A. F. The American Nurses Association and Continuing Education. In *Critical Issues in Continuing Education,* pp. 71–78. National Conference on Continuing Education in Nursing, University of Wisconsin in Madison, Wisconsin, 1971.
3. "Continuing Education Working Statement," p. 2. A Joint Statement of the Task Force on Revision of the Model Law of the ANA Congress for Nursing Practice and the Interim Executive Committee of the ANA Council on Continuing Education, American Nurses Association, Kansas City, Missouri, May 1973, 8 pp. mimeo.
4. "An Interim Statement on Continuing Education in Nursing." Guidelines prepared by the Organizing Group for the ANA Council on Continuing Education and released for circulation by the ANA Commission on Education, American Nurses Association, Kansas City, Missouri, September 1972, mimeo.
5. *Ibid,* p. 1.
6. McNally, J. M. *Continuing Education For Nurses: A Survey of Current Programs.* Kansas City, Mo.: American Nurses Association, 1972.
7. National University Extension Association, *op. cit.*
8. *Statement of Interpretation and Clarification on the Use of C.E.U.* Interim Executive Committee for ANA Council on Continuing Education for Nursing. Kansas City, Mo.: American Nurses Association, May 2, 1973, p. 1.
9. *Ibid,* p. 2.
10. Knowles, M. S. *The Modern Practice of Adult Education.* New York: Association Press, 1970, p. 22.
11. Houle, C. O. The Comparative Study of Continuing Professional Education. *J. Continuing Ed. Nurs.* 3:4, 1972.
12. McNally, J. M. *op cit.,* p. 49.

What About the CEU?

by MARJORIE MOORE CANTOR

This is the fourth article by **Marjorie Moore Cantor** appearing in this reader. This article is reprinted from JONA, September-October, 1974.

Whether we like it or not, we have to contend with the issue of continuing education documentation for registered nurses. Although such documentation may be a hasty solution to a problem that has not been clearly identified, the trend toward emphasis on continuing education programming seems inexorable. Even if a given state does not make continuing education experiences a prerequisite for relicensure, it seems likely that there will be pressure from other sources for nurses to provide documentation of such experiences, whether by CEU (continuing education units) or some other means of certification. It is also likely that the employing agency will be expected to assist the registered nurse in obtaining the education, though ostensibly it is the responsibility of the individual nurse to do so.

Mandatory continuing education and the meaning of the CEU have been well handled by others [1-4]. What has not been discussed in any detail are the implications this movement has for institutions and inference on the staff development programs of nursing departments. Few of the existing continuing education programs have originated out of a careful identification of health care problems. Methods for determining what content is needed are extremely primitive in most cases. Some programs were developed on the basis of an analysis of patient needs and an identification of the nursing skills required to assure competency in a given practice area, but these are the exceptions. Important names and currently popular nursing fads most often constitute the basis for the selection of continuing education offerings. A perusal of the numerous brochures that come across one's desk each week indicates that we tend to dabble in the various popular topics of the day instead of determining what constitutes the most meaningful content required to meet the obligations of our departments. A director of nursing contributes to this proliferation of useless programs when she rewards staff for the accumulation of CEU's without considering the ultimate effects of the experience on patient care or when she depends on others to make important decisions about the learning needs of her staff. So does she also when she fails to determine if the existing structure for accrediting continuing education programs is contributing to better programs. Those of us (inservice educators, continuing education faculties) who are responsible for preparing individuals to perform particular services need validation from practice areas that what we are doing is achieving the purpose at hand.

Because we have a vested interest in perpetuating our own methods and content, and because we ourselves do not use the services of those whom we train, we are disqualified as the final judges of the adequacy of our work. The question of who *is* qualified to judge such work is not an easy one to answer. But we must find a better answer than we now have if continuing education is to have a beneficial impact on the health delivery system. Current methods of evaluating educational programs by examining their content and structure without reference to what the program is supposed to achieve in the way of improving patient care, are not bringing us nearer to well-prepared practitioners.

The ultimate outcome of this concentration on the process instead of on the results to be accomplished is that the structure for accrediting programs becomes more complex and restrictive. Agreed, standards must be set up to protect the consumer and to eliminate the specious and the fraudulent programs. But it is possible to set up structures for establishing standards and approval systems that protect the self-interest of the educational groups in question and do nothing to contribute to the welfare of the consumer. Under certain CEU approval systems, for example, a nurse in an isolated community who does not control the temperature of a high risk infant, with the consequence that the ailing infant's survival chances are remote, could satisfy her relicensure requirements by attending a conference on parenting techniques or child development concepts for nurses, content not very pertinent to the needs of that unfortunate infant. Whether any system could eliminate all such abuses is questionable, but groups concerned with continuing education should at least try to come to grips with existing realities before establishing an approval system.

Those directing and accountable for nursing care programs are the persons who must provide the information needed to determine if existing systems of continuing education result in improvement of quality care without an undue financial burden being imposed on the patient as a result. These individuals can inhibit or foster the staff's participation in CEU gathering in which everyone considers that her obligation regarding self-development has been met either by presenting a continuing education program or by attending one, regardless of its relevance.

We cannot expect that the needed control will be exerted by nurses in general, nor can we expect them to be rational about the significance of continuing education as a means of improving quality care when the system itself fosters irrationality. The demands by nurses to receive credit for whatever lecture, class, or organizational meeting they choose to attend and their selections of content on the basis of potential ''credit'' to be received for the work rather than on its pertinence to their jobs are to be expected. The assumptions that the CEU necessarily has some kind of significance and that built-in ''protection'' exists by virtue of the assignment of CEU credit are bound to be instilled in nurses when all programs include a statement about CEU in their advance announcements and various agencies and institutions vie for approval rights. The idea that approval by one group does not guarantee acceptance of the credit on the part of another group fails to enter into the thinking of either the organization providing the program or the individuals who are its consumers.

It is important for directors of nursing to insist that their standards for quality care be met and that continuing education be directed to the goal of providing staff the information and skills needed to make it possible to meet these care standards. The most critical basis for approving or disapproving a continuing educational offering for credit by any group should be evidence provided by that group documenting *the relationship of the program's content to specific problems of patient care delivery formulated in patient care terms.* This evidence serves as an accomplished ultimate result.

It has been argued that this degree of specificity is not possible, that there is no way to be certain that a given educational program will have its intended effect. At a minimum, a group seeking to sell educational offerings should be able to describe the basis on which it was decided that its offerings are needed, the health care problem involved, the program content directly related to its solution, and the level at which the program can be provided. Undoubtedly, these bases would eliminate many of the current continuing education topics and would reduce the number of programs that would receive accreditation.

At the individual department level, there are relevant planning issues. We need to develop workable methods by which all staff members will be prepared to meet relicensing requirements that are likely to be imposed by the state, while at the same time making certain that existing staff development programs, specific to the needs of the patients in that institution, are not sacrificed in the process. Although the director of nursing may believe she is not obligated to arrange for her staff to meet the requirements of some other state or the criteria of groups other than the licensing agency, she is likely to find that pressures from both within and outside her staff and institution make it impossible to ignore these considerations. She must also take into account the cost to the patient and the potential problems that may be created by staff release time and the attendant reduction in available personnel. Thus, decisions about ways to solve the problem of enabling staff to accumulate educational experience must be made scrupulously if the director is neither to increase the cost of staffing unduly nor penalize and antagonize her staff members.

Careful planning calls for, more than anything else, knowledge on the part of the director of nursing about what is going to make a difference to patients. If she is developing quality assurance programs using patient outcome criteria, as is now being required by the Joint Commission for Accreditation of Hospitals, she will have such knowledge. Other systems of evaluation have tended to focus on the nursing process; the use of patient-outcome criteria provides a much better picture of the content required. When she has this information at hand, she can communicate it to the groups that will be making decisions about educational programs and she can use it to set priorities for her own department's system.

The first priority for support ought to focus on those programs that are directly related to the needs of the departmental staff at all levels of functioning. If the resources required for these purposes are available within the local community, then establishing programs in that setting will provide the most economical way to educate large groups of individuals. If these local programs can gain approval from the appropriate accrediting group, they will serve the additional role of providing a way for staff to accumulate credit. To make it possible for local agencies to receive approval for their educational offerings, it is important that the credit approving groups not make the requirements so restrictive that only programs offered within a formal educational setting or taught by members of nursing faculties could qualify. A requirement of the nursing department that internal continuing education programs meet the same criteria as would be required by the director of nursing for external offerings would constitute a first step toward providing programs that would permit both the acquisition of needed skills and the fulfillment of qualifications for relicensure.

Some content needed to improve the care delivery system and the program of care for a group of patients undoubtedly would not be obtainable in the local community. These cases would require educational leave for selected staff members who could then participate in relevant programs offered elsewhere. If the sequence of planning moves from educational needs to educational programs, rather than in the opposite direction, it is likely that the nursing leadership group will tend to be more responsible than they were previously in requesting departmental support for staff education programs. The fact that something is available would cease to be a basis for incorporating it into the staff development program.

A carefully planned internal staff education program can provide staff with the opportunity to acquire needed continuing education credits. But it would probably also be wise to provide for a *minimal* amount of educational leave time to allow the individual staff member to further her own personal career plans, the only restriction being that it be used just for educational programs and conferences at a time that would not jeopardize the ongoing patient care program. Given a standard amount of time for individualized, outside experiences, it would then be possible to restrict department-supported educational programs to those that are relevant to existing departmental needs.

To impress on staff that the purpose of obtaining additional education is to improve the quality of patient care, the department can selectively approve credits achieved by staff on the basis of the content's potential for preparing them for promotion. It is also important to help staff realize that they must invest something of themselves in return for educational credit and that this investment should include the achievement of new skills, rather than just the passive assimilation of content.

If leaders in the practice setting are going to be able to satisfy demands that they insure the competency of the professional nursing care given to the consumer, they will have to abandon their blind faith in the effectiveness of unselected educational programs and on the wisdom of educators in determining what is needed by the staff members responsible for giving daily patient care. The continuing education groups (both within and outside of nursing), the nurse speciality groups, the colleges and universities, the state nursing associations, the legislatures, and the licensing boards are all indicating that they know the educational needs of nurses, but the members of these groups do not have to confront the patients who have not received adequate nursing care: Should not the directors of nursing at least make certain that these groups be provided the significant, relevant information about the nursing aspects of the health delivery system?

REFERENCES

1. Gwaltney, B. H. The continuing education unit, *Nurs. Outlook*, 21:500, 1973.
2. Hatfield, P. Mandatory continuing education, *JONA*, 6:35, 1973.
3. Hornbeck, M. S. Measuring continuing education, *Am. J. Nurs*, 73:1576, 1973.
4. Stevens, B.J. Mandatory continuing education for professional nurse relicensure: What are the issues? *JONA*, 5:24, 1973.